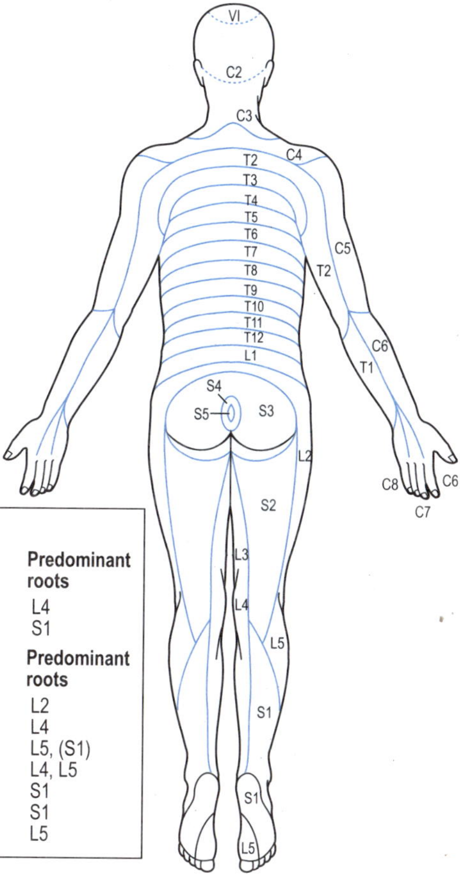

LOWER LIMB

Reflexes	**Predominant roots**
Knee	L4
Ankle	S1
Major motor groups	**Predominant roots**
Hip flexion	L2
Knee extension	L4
Knee flexion	L5, (S1)
Ankle dorsiflexion	L4, L5
Ankle plantar flexion	S1
Eversion of ankle	S1
Inversion of ankle	L5

Approximate distribution of dermatomes, with root values of reflexes and major motor groups

CHURCHILL'S POCKETBOOK OF
Pain

This book is dedicated to our husbands and children without whose support and sacrifice it could not have been written

For Churchill Livingstone

Publisher: Michael Parkinson
Project Editor: Janice Urquhart
Copy Editor: Jennifer Bew
Indexer: Liza Weinkove
Design Direction: Erik Bigland
Project Controller: Nancy Arnott
Page Layout: Kate Walshaw

CHURCHILL'S POCKETBOOK OF Pain

Catherine F. Stannard FRCA
Consultant in Pain Management and Anaesthesia,
Frenchay Hospital, Bristol, UK

Sara Booth FFARCSI
Health Services Fellow and Consultant
Physician in Palliative Medicine (Research),
Sir Michael Sobell House, Oxford, UK

With contributions by
Chris Eccleston PhD
Director, Pain Management Unit,
Royal National Hospital for Rheumatic Diseases,
Bath and University of Bath, UK

Tim Cook FRCA
Specialist Registrar, Bristol School of Anaesthesia, UK

Illustrated by
Robert Britton

CHURCHILL LIVINGSTONE

EDINBURGH LONDON NEW YORK PHILADELPHIA
SAN FRANCISCO SYDNEY TORONTO 1998

CHURCHILL LIVINGSTONE
A Division of Harcourt Brace and Company Limited

Robert Stevenson House
1–3 Baxter's Place
Leith Walk
Edinburgh
EH1 3AF

First published 1998

ISBN 0 443 05322 7

British Library Cataloguing in Publication Data
A catalogue record for this book is available from the British Library.

Library of Congress Cataloging in Publication Data
A catalog record for this book is available from the Library of Congress.

Produced by Addison Wesley Longman Singapore Pte Ltd
Printed in Singapore

Preface

The management of pain is poorly taught and misconceptions abound. In particular the management of chronic pain seems mysterious and its scientific basis unclear. This pocketbook attempts to draw aside the veil and reveal the rationale as well as the practical conduct of pain management.

This is not intended as a comprehensive textbook, but is designed to fit easily into a pocket or briefcase to provide a readily accessible overview of the aetiology and management of common painful conditions. The first section of the book describes the science on which the practice of pain management is based. The next three sections describe common conditions encountered in clinical practice and necessarily reflect the clinical experience of the authors. The psychology of pain management is discussed in section 5, but it is important to realise that this underpins all pain therapy described in earlier chapters.

Much of pain management, especially in the field of chronic pain is based on accumulated clinical experience albeit with scientific basis. Systematic reviews are already guiding us along the most appropriate pathways for management and will do so increasingly, however, this book is based on current common clinical practice.

This book will be useful to trainees in palliative care and pain management, particularly in their attachments to a pain clinic. In addition we hope that experienced clinicians in these fields will find information of interest within its pages. The regular activities of many other disciplines (who do not receive formal training in pain control) include the management of both acute and chronic pain and this book, whilst not intended as a 'do it yourself' guide' should aid logical practice.

Catherine F. Stannard — Bristol
Sara Booth — Oxford
1997

Acknowledgements

Sara Booth would like to express her gratitude for the time spent by busy eminent colleagues in reading and commenting on her script particularly Dame Cicely Saunders, Drs John Reynolds, Chris Glynn, Tim Jack, Michael O'Connor, Elaine Sugden and Mary Miller.

Cathy Stannard is indebted to Dr Di Brighouse for her comments and advice on the essentials of obstetric pain management, Mr George Malcolm of the Department of Neurosurgery at Frenchay Hospital for bringing order and clarity to the jungle of back pain management, Christine Dyer, physiotherapist for her practical and experienced help in the field of TENS and Rose Moreton for her help in preparation of artwork.

We are grateful for the support of the staff at Churchill Livingstone in particular Janice Urquhart our project editor.

Contents

SECTION 1

PRINCIPLES OF PAIN MANAGEMENT

CHAPTER 1

ANATOMY AND PHYSIOLOGY OF PAIN

Pain is a complex sensory and emotional experience which is integrated at the level of the cerebral cortex, and the signal that is interpreted as pain can arise at any point in the pain pathway. However, the route by which a noxious stimulus gives rise to the experience of pain can be considered anatomically. The 'physical' way in which we feel pain can be considered under a number of headings:

- Peripheral receptors
- Primary afferent conduction
- Dorsal horn
- Ascending tracts and cortical projections
- Descending modulation of pain
- Visceral pain, role of autonomic nervous system (ANS)
- Chemicals involved in pain transmission
- Response of nervous system to injury

Peripheral receptors

Painful (tissue-damaging) stimuli activate specific pain receptors (nociceptors) in the tissues, which transform pain information into an electrical signal which is conducted centrally. These are the free nerve endings of unmyelinated and finely myelinated neurones, and are of two types. One group respond to mechanical deformation and are described as high-threshold mechanoreceptors (HTM); the others respond to a variety of noxious inputs and are polymodal nociceptors (PMN). A number of chemicals are involved in stimulation and sensitization of PMNs, including hydrogen ions, bradykinin, histamine, prostaglandins, leucotrienes 5HT and cytokines. The receptors (and the fibres of which they are the free nerve endings) have a number of properties, summarized in Table 1.1.

TABLE 1.1 Characteristics of primary afferent fibres

Fibre type	*A δ (finely myelinated)*	*C (unmyelinated)*
Fibre diameter	2–5 μm	<2 μm
Conduction velocity	5–15 ms^{-1}	0.5–2 ms^{-1}
Distribution	Body surface, muscles, joints	Most tissues
Pain to which stimulation leads	Rapid, pricking, well localised	Slow, diffuse, dull, aching

Primary afferent conduction

Nociceptor terminations join to form axons, whose cell bodies are in the dorsal root ganglia or trigeminal ganglion. The characteristics of these axons have been outlined in Table 1.1 The central terminations of these fibres are in the dorsal horn of the spinal cord (Figure 1.1) The majority enter the dorsal horn in the ventrolateral bundle of the dorsal root (lateral to the larger-diameter myelinated Aβ fibres). However, about 30% of the central processes of unmyelinated fibres enter the spinal cord through the ventral root, although they too terminate in the dorsal horn of the cord. On entering the cord the roots may bifurcate into ascending and descending branches, which may enter the dorsal horn one or two segments above or below the segment of origin.

Dorsal horn of spinal cord

The dorsal horns of the cord are divided into (Rexed) laminae on the basis of their histological appearances. There are numerous connections between the laminae, although they do have discrete functions related to pain processing. Lamina II, the substantia gelatinosa, extends from the trigeminal nucleus in the medulla to the filum terminale. C fibres terminate in lamina II. Aδ fibres terminate in laminae I and V. Aβ fibres, which respond to innocuous stimuli such as vibration and light touch, enter the cord medial to the dorsal horn and pass without synapse to the dorsal columns; however, they give off collateral branches to the dorsal horn which terminate in several laminae, particularly III–V and deeper. They also synapse directly with terminals of unmyelinated C fibres in lamina II. The laminae that receive afferent input from both large- and small-diameter fibres (i.e. II and V) are important sites for pain modulation and localization. From lamina III and deeper, information is summated from direct input from the periphery and from more dorsal laminae.

The extent to which painful peripheral stimuli are conducted centrally (and perceived as pain) depends upon the degree to which two major modulating mechanisms at the level of the dorsal horn 'close the gate' to onward transmission (Figure 1.2):

1. Activity in large myelinated afferent (Aβ) fibres is via inhibitory circuits in the superficial laminae of the dorsal horn to suppress transmission in small unmyelinated (C fibre) afferents.
2. Inhibitory control from higher centres is tonically active (see overleaf).

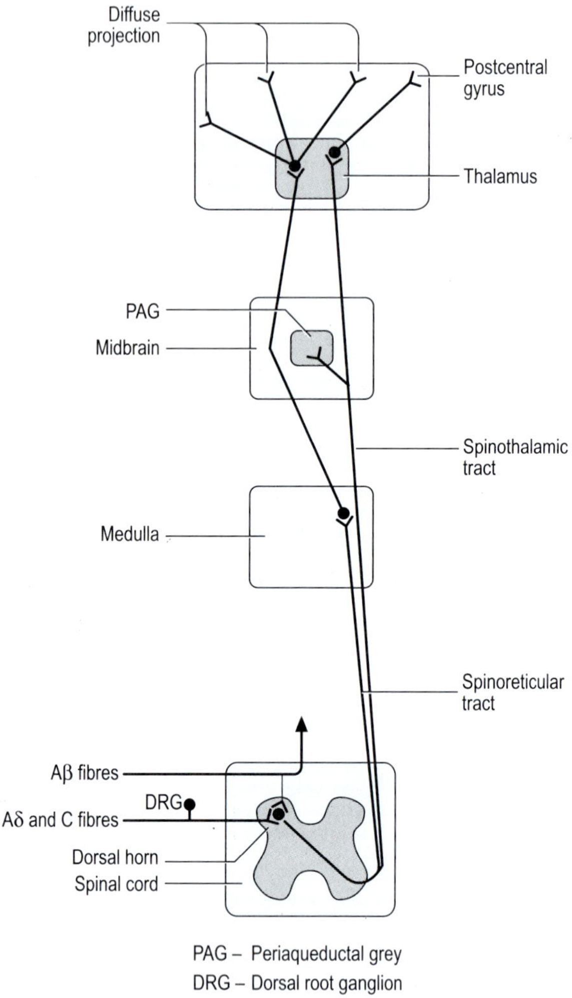

A

Fig. 1.1 Schematic representation of (**A**) ascending and (**B**) descending pain pathways.

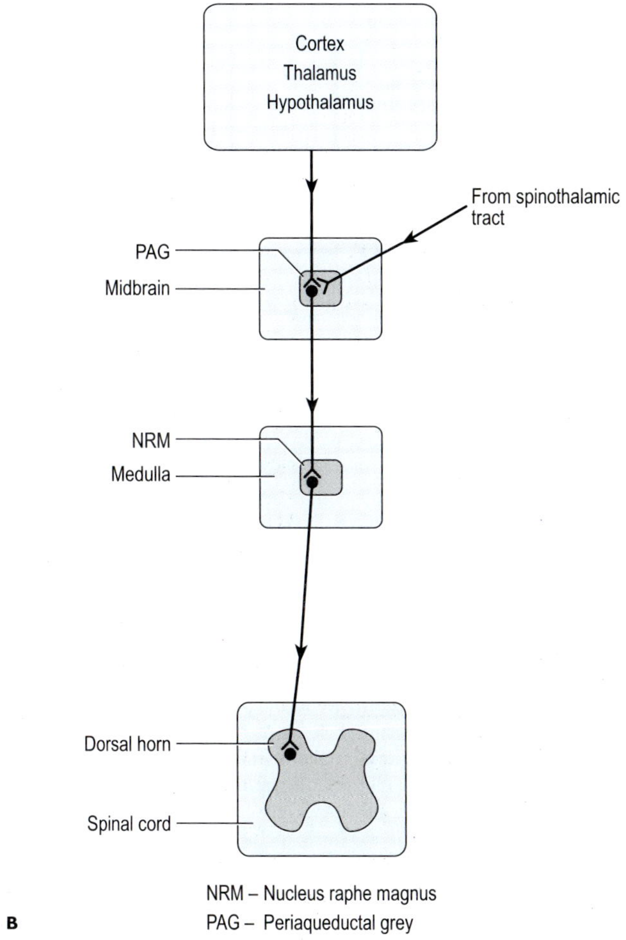
Cortex
Thalamus
Hypothalamus
From spinothalamic tract
PAG
Midbrain
NRM
Medulla
Dorsal horn
Spinal cord
NRM – Nucleus raphe magnus
PAG – Periaqueductal grey
B

Fig. 1.1 (**B**)

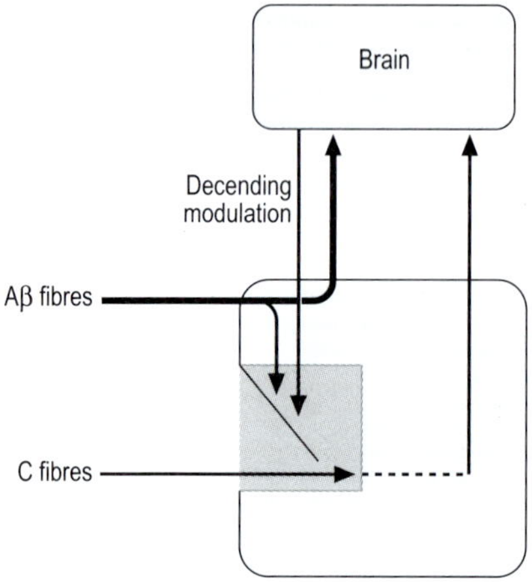

Fig. 1.2 Schematic representation of dorsal horn 'gating' mechanism. The onward transmission of nociceptive (C fibre) activity is determined by the degree to which the dorsal horn 'gate' is open. The gate may be shut by activity in Aβ collaterals and by descending modulation.

Ascending tracts

From the dorsal horn, nociceptor neurones ascend in the contralateral spinothalamic and spinoreticular tracts in the anterolateral white matter of the spinal cord. The spinothalamic tract is the more recently evolved, and principally comprises axons of neurones in laminae I and V of the dorsal horn, in which most Aδ fibres terminate. These ascend to the ventral posterior lateral nucleus of the thalamus and thence to the postcentral gyrus. Axons are somatotopically organized, with caudal elements found laterally to those from more rostral structures. The spinothalamic tract sends collateral branches to the periaqueductal grey (PAG) matter in the midbrain (see below).

The more (phylogenetically) ancient spinoreticular pathway arises from cells deeper in the grey matter of the dorsal horn, including lamina V (it should be remembered that these laminae receive inputs from more dorsal laminae, e.g. II, via several interneurones). Fibres ascend in the anterolateral cord and reach the nuclei of the brainstem reticular formation, whence they project to the thalamus, hypothalamus and thalamic intralaminar nuclei. These latter project diffusely to the whole cerebral cortex. This system shows little somatotopic organization and is involved in the perception of diffuse, emotionally disturbing pain.

Descending modulation of pain (Figure 1.1B)

Electrical stimulation of the midbrain PAG produces profound analgesia. During stimulation, responses to non-noxious stimuli remain normal and subjects are alert. Injection of morphine to this region produces a greater analgesic effect than at any other site in the CNS. The PAG receives input from the thalamus, hypothalamus, the cortex and collaterals from the spinothalamic tract, and so is an important centre for descending control of pain. The PAG projects to the nucleus raphe magnus in the medulla. Axons from this nucleus descend in the dorsolateral funiculus of the spinal cord to the dorsal horn.

Brainstem neurones may control nociceptive transmission by:

- direct action on dorsal horn cells
- inhibition of excitatory dorsal horn neurones
- excitation of inhibitory neurones.

Such descending inhibitory activity may explain why **emotions** and **behaviour** can influence pain.

Visceral pain

Pain arising from viscera has a number of features which distinguish it from the somatic pain described above. It is:

- Poorly localized
- Associated with nausea and autonomic disturbance
- Maybe colicky, i.e. spasmodic in nature
- Often referred to another part of the body
- Stimuli that cause somatic pain, e.g. cutting, crushing, are not painful when applied to viscera. Pain is elicited by distension, ischaemia and inflammation.

Pain is mediated via Aδ and C fibres, which travel with autonomic afferents that enter the spinal cord at the thoracic, upper lumbar and sacral segments. The incoming afferents give off collaterals which travel up and down the cord and penetrate the grey matter in laminae I and V. Transmission onwards from the spinal cord is in the same ascending tracts as somatic information. Because pathways are shared, activity in postsynaptic cells produced by visceral afferent activity is interpreted as arising from converging somatic afferents, and pain may be referred to the corresponding somatic tissue.

Role of the sympathetic nervous system

The sympathetic nervous system is involved in the genesis and maintenance of a number of painful conditions (see Complex regional pain syndrome, Chapter 19). Following injury, particularly to a limb, there is abnormal activity and sensitization of primary afferents, which in turn leads to abnormal processing of information in the spinal cord. This is associated with abnormal sympathetic outflow to the injured extremity, which leads to:

- abnormal regulation of vasculature
- oedema
- discoloration
- changes in sweating
- temperature changes
- trophic changes in the skin
- reduced motor activity in the affected part.

Sympathetic noradrenergic neurones can influence nociceptive primary afferents. The chemical influence of noradrenaline can be exerted at nerve terminals, along the axon or in the dorsal root ganglion. One of the neural responses to injury is the increased expression of α-adrenoceptors in nociceptive neurones. Some of the effects of sympathetic nerves on primary afferents may be mediated by alteration in the blood supply to afferent nerve terminals.

Chemicals involved in nociception

A large number of substances are involved in pain appreciation, and knowledge of their actions forms the basis of a number of pain therapies. Some of the important chemicals are described in Table 1.2.

How the nervous system alters in response to injury

The nervous system is not hard wired: it changes its structure and function in response to the input it receives, i.e. it is plastic. Plasticity is evident at all levels, from the nociceptor to the cortex. Peripherally nociceptors can be sensitized by injury, decreasing their threshold and increasing their response to noxious stimuli. In addition they become sensitive to non-noxious stimuli. When an axon is cut, the proximal end forms a swelling or neuroma. Neuromata may also form if a nerve is partially damaged. Spontaneous electrical activity has been demonstrated in neuromata and damaged nerves which may be due to alteration in the quantity and distribution of ion channel protein. The rate of ectopic firing is influenced by physical stimuli (heat, cold etc.) and the metabolic and chemical environment of the nerve and by sympathetic efferent activity. These peripheral changes are accompanied by central sensitization. It can be shown in the dorsal horn of the cord that repetitive C-fibre activation leads to an augmented response to subsequent C-fibre input: so-called 'wind-up'. Central sensitization is characterized by enhanced transmission of nociceptive information, sensitivity to non-nociceptive inputs and spontaneous impulse generation in the spinal cord. The neurochemistry of these central changes is similar to that of memory, and involves NMDA and nitric oxide.

TABLE 1.2 Important chemicals involved in nociception

Substance	*Comments*
Amines	
Noradrenaline	Involved in descending modulation of pain, probably acts via α_2 receptors
Serotonin	Involved in descending modulation of pain – all 5HT receptor subtypes probably involved
Endogenous opioid peptides	
Enkephalins *β-Endorphin* *Dynorphins*	Derived from biologically inactive peptide precursors produced in cell body of neurone and transported to axon terminal. Distributed widely in CNS but particularly in sites associated with pain. Act as endogenous ligands for opioid receptors (μ, δ and κ). Produce primary inhibitory effects.
Non-opioid peptides	
Substance P	Widespread in nociceptive pathways, particularly DRG of C fibres and C fibre central terminations. Release induces signs of inflammation.
Cholecystokinin, angiotensin II, oxytocin, somatostatin, VIP	Occur in DRG, dorsal horn and spinal tracts involved in pain. May be involved in perception of visceral pain. Nerve injury causes depletion of these substances in dorsal horn.
Excitatory amino acids	
Glutamate *Aspartate*	Act on *N*-methyl-D-aspartate (NMDA) and non-NMDA receptors. Involved in development, memory and neuronal plasticity.
Inhibitory amino acids	
GABA *Glycine*	Regulate behaviour generated by non-noxious stimuli e.g. low-threshold afferent transmission by tonic activity in GABAergic and glycinergic neurones. Antagonists to these substances lead to pain behaviour following innocuous stimuli.
Nitric oxide (NO)	NO synthesized from L-arginine by NO synthase present in sensory neurones and dorsal horn. Involved in peripheral and central sensitization in response to injury and linked with NMDA activity.

CHAPTER 2

CLINICAL PHARMACOLOGY

DEFINITIONS OF PHARMACOLOGICAL TERMS

This section gives a brief overview of some pharmacological principles. First, some key terms are defined and the available routes for drug administration reviewed: an understanding of these helps in assessing the usefulness of a drug for a clinical situation. The pharmacology of the most commonly used drugs in pain therapy is outlined in the chapters that follow.

Opioid

This refers to any substance that binds specifically to endogenous opioid receptors and produces some agonist activity, i.e. it has 'morphine-like' activity. 'Endogenous' used in this context means receptors found **within** the body. A drug classified as an opioid does not necessarily have the same pharmacological profile as morphine. Opioids are neurotransmitters and neurohormones in a complex signalling system which produces both inhibition (in the spinal cord this results in an analgesic effect) and stimulation (in the chemoreceptor trigger zone this produces nausea and vomiting).

Opiate was the word used for a drug derived from the opium poppy (*Papaver somniferum*), for example morphine. 'Opioid' now embraces this group of drugs as well as synthetic opioids.

Opioid receptors

Opioids, both endogenous and exogenous, act by binding with specific opioid receptors. Three opioid receptors have been described – μ, δ and κ – and all are involved in analgesia. They are listed in Table 2.1. These opioid receptors

TABLE 2.1 Opioid receptors

Receptor	*Endogenous ligand*	*Exogenous ligand**	*Actions*
μ	β-Endorphin Enkephalins	Fentanyl Morphine	Analgesia Respiratory depression Euphoria Dependence
κ	Dynorphins		Spinal analgesia Sedation Miosis
δ	Enkephalins		Analgesia Respiratory depression Euphoria Constipation Motivation, arousal, learning† Stress response to pain Immunomodulation

* ligand, a substance which binds to a receptor. It may act as an agonist or an antagonist.
† this is still an unconfirmed research finding

are found at high concentrations throughout the central nervous system (CNS), but they are also found peripherally. Most work on their exact localization has been done on animal preparations and may not always be relevant to humans. It is well known that the laboratory pharmacology of opioids, on pain-free volunteers, is different from the effects seen when morphine is used clinically.

Endogenous opioids

These are the peptides produced by the body which have morphine-like properties. Three distinct families, from different precursors, have been described and are shown in Table 2.2.

TABLE 2.2 Endogenous opioids

Opioid	*Precursor*
Endorphins	Preopiomelanocortin
Enkephalins	Preproenkephalin
Dynorphins	Preprodynorphin

Although there is some relationship between these families and the actions produced at the specific receptors listed above, endogenous opioids are not specific for a single type of receptor. All are produced by a common mechanism:

gene induction ⇒ mRNA production ⇒ precursor polypeptide ⇒ post-translational processing ⇒ final peptide (the endogenous opioid).

The individual endogenous opioids are produced in different quantities under different conditions.

Exogenous opioids

These are the administered drugs, such as morphine, which bind to opioid receptors to produce analgesia and other effects.

Receptor agonist

A drug which binds to a receptor and stimulates it. A full agonist will stimulate the receptor to its maximum extent. Morphine is such a drug, acting mainly at the μ receptor to produce strong analgesia.

Receptor antagonist

A drug which binds to a receptor, preventing other drugs from so doing, and which does not stimulate the receptor at all. Naloxone is a opioid receptor antagonist and reverses the effects of morphine. A pure antagonist has no activity of its own and 'needs' the presence of an endogenous agonist to show an effect.

Partial agonist

A drug which binds to a receptor but does not produce maximum stimulation. Because it occupies the receptor it can prevent a concurrently administered agonist with weaker receptor affinity from producing its full effect, and so acts like a partial antagonist. Buprenorphine is a partial μ agonist. A partial agonist will not produce the same analgesia as a pure agonist at any dose – it will not be as efficacious, and this implies that there will be a ceiling to its analgesic effect. In theory, the administration of morphine and buprenorphine simultaneously to the same patient should reduce the efficacy of morphine; in practice this antagonism only seems to occur when high doses are used. It is clearly best not to prescribe both drugs at the same time, so that unintended antagonism cannot occur.

Mixed agonists–antagonists

Mixed agonists–anatagonists act simultaneously at the different receptor subtypes with a mixture of agonist and antagonist actions. Pentazocine is an example of such a drug, having agonist activity at κ receptors, partial μ agonism and δ antagonism. Such drugs tend to have a lower dependency potential.

Potency

This reflects the dose of a drug needed to produce a given effect – it is related to the degree of attraction between a drug and its receptor. Dextropropoxyphene, a weak opioid and a component of coproxamol, is a weak analgesic because it has a weak affinity for the μ receptor.

Efficacy

Efficacy is related to the power of a drug to achieve an outcome. At the level of the receptor, morphine is a more effective μ agonist than buprenorphine, which is only a partial agonist: there is a ceiling to the analgesia possible with buprenorphine, however high a dose is given. At the level of the whole organism, the efficacy of a drug is more complex and is a reflection of the ability of the drug to achieve an effect such as analgesia or antiemesis; a drug–receptor interaction starts the process but many other interactions and pathways may then be involved. There are also pharmacokinetic differences between drugs, which sometimes mean that the efficacy of the drug at receptor level is not translated into efficacy in the whole animal.

The ceiling effect

This refers to the phenomenon that there is a limit to the degree of pain relief that many drugs can give, however high a dose is used. This is influenced by two pharmacodynamic factors:

- Agonist activity, as described for buprenorphine, above
- The incidence of adverse effects: for example, the analgesic activity of codeine in clinical practice is restricted by the unacceptable frequency of nausea, vomiting and constipation as the dose is increased; similarly, pethidine should not be used in chronic pain, or in high doses, as a toxic metabolite – norpethidine – accumulates, causing convulsions.

Dependency

A person is dependent on an opioid when its sudden absence produces a physical withdrawal syndrome. An addict is one who uses a drug for recreational purposes and suffers both physical and psychological symptoms when the drug is stopped. Withdrawal is so intolerable that an addict will do almost anything to maintain a supply. Addiction is so rare when opioids are taken for medical reasons that it should not influence prescribing in all but the most high-risk patients.

Tolerance

Tolerance is present when increasing doses of a drug are needed to produce the same pharmacological effect. In the management of cancer pain it has been shown that when an increase in dose is needed it is usually because the disease is progressing, not because the patient is becoming tolerant to morphine. In clinical practice the dangers of tolerance and dependency have been exaggerated, which has worked against good pain relief for many people and led to unnecessary suffering. Both tolerance and dependency are more likely to develop when a drug is used intravenously.

Tolerance to the different pharmacological effects of a drug develops at different rates: for example, most patients become tolerant to the sedating or emetic effects of morphine within a few days of starting it, and yet never become tolerant to its constipating effect.

The World Health Organization (WHO) analgesic ladder (Figure 2.1)

This is a tool developed by the WHO as a guide to pharmacological therapy for cancer and other chronic pain. Drug treatment is now the cornerstone of cancer pain management: 70–90% of patients can obtain adequate pain relief from analgesic drugs alone. A further 20% will require additional interventions. The ladder suggests a stepwise approach to drug therapy depending on the severity of the pain. If the pain is mild a non-opioid such as paracetamol can be given regularly: if this is not sufficient, a Step 2 drug (e.g. a weak opioid) should be taken regularly. If the pain is still poorly controlled or disease

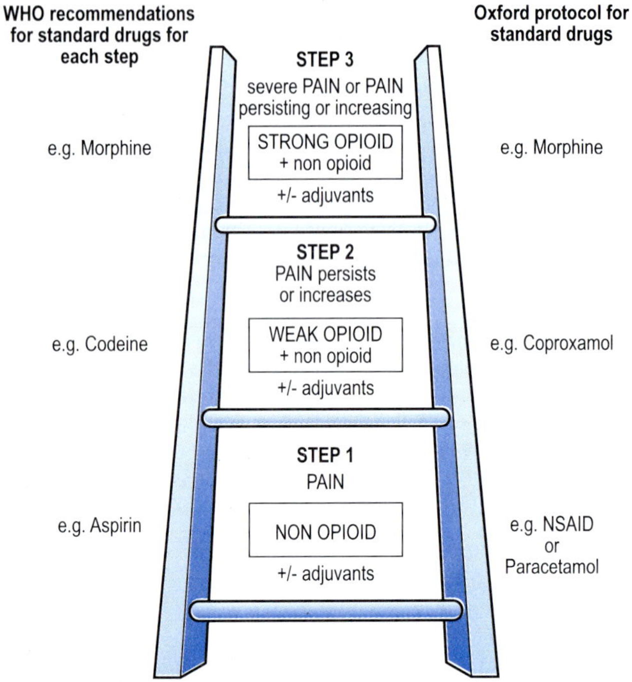

Fig. 2.1 The WHO analgesic ladder for cancer and other chronic pain.

progression has occurred and the pain has intensified, then a Step 3 drug, e.g. morphine, should be administered regularly. At every step adjuvant (see below) drug therapy may be needed. When a patient moves up the ladder the non-opioid is often continued with benefit. The ladder is both an educational tool and a guideline for treatment, and it has been demonstrated to improve cancer pain management in centres where treatment was previously unstructured. If the patient is in severe pain at the first assessment the clinician should obviously use a Step 3 drug as first-line management, and **titrate the dose against the pain**. Pain therapy needs constant review, particularly in a condition such as cancer, where the disease may be constantly changing.

Adjuvant drugs

These may be used in pain therapy:

- to counter the adverse effects of an analgesic drug: for example the use of laxatives when opioids are prescribed
- as co-analgesics: for example dexamethasone may be used to reduce oedema round a tumour, so reducing pressure on an adjacent nerve
- as psychotropic medication: for example the treatment of depression in a cancer patient or one with chronic pain
- as analgesics in their own right: for example the use of an antidepressant or anticonvulsant in neuropathic pain.

ROUTES OF ADMINISTRATION

Oral absorption

This is the commonest route of drug administration and is to be preferred wherever possible; it is the simplest, least hazardous, most convenient and cheapest of all the possible ways of administering medication.

A drug will only be absorbed from the gastrointestinal tract (GI) when it is in a unionized state. Aspirin, which is acidic, is absorbed in the acid environment of the stomach, but most drugs are absorbed in the small intestine.

Other factors affecting oral absorption are:

- Stomach contents: fatty meals and antacids delay drug absorption
- Gastric motility: opioids, for example, inhibit gastric emptying and most drugs are absorbed in the small intestine, therefore drug absorption is slowed
- low splanchnic blood flow: this is markedly reduced in hypovolaemia, and so is drug absorption
- drug formulation: the size of drug particle and its pH will affect its absorption.

Figure 2.2 illustrates the effect of drug formulation on absorption using aspirin as an example.

First-pass metabolism (presystemic metabolism)

After a drug is absorbed from the gut it must pass through the liver before reaching the systemic circulation; it will be metabolized to a greater or lesser extent during this process. A drug such as naloxone is almost entirely inactivated on this journey, and is said to undergo complete first-pass metabolism. It is impractical to administer drugs like this by mouth: they are said to have a large oral to parenteral ratio. For naloxone the oral to parenteral ratio is 50:1, indicating that in order to give an equivalent dose by mouth 50 times the parenteral dose would have to be given.

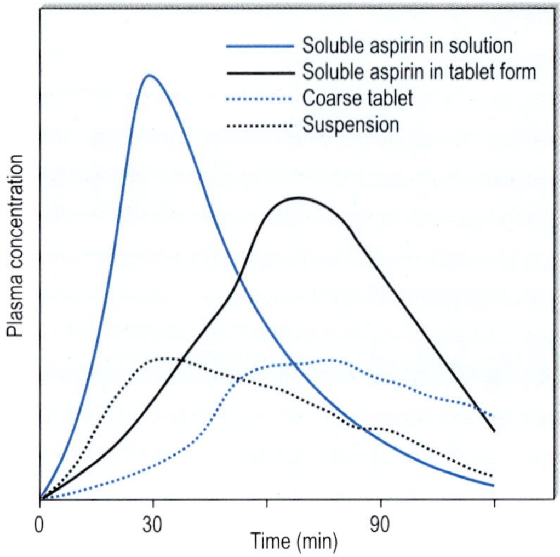

Fig. 2.2 Influence of drug formulation on absorption of aspirin (acetylsalicylic acid). (Modified from Kaufman L, Jahemer PV 1996 Pharmacology in the practice of anaesthesia. Edward Arnold, with permission.)

The extent of first-pass metabolism with a given drug may vary greatly between individuals, and this partly accounts for the huge range of doses of the same drug needed by different patients. This is observed with oral morphine. Bioavailability is the fraction of a drug that is pharmacologically active after oral absorption compared with that achieved by i.v. administration.

ALTERNATIVE ROUTES OF ADMINISTRATION

Most of the time it is safest, easiest and most comfortable to administer drugs by mouth, but this may be impossible for reasons related to the patient's condition, the illness being treated or the drug being used. Alternative routes of administration are discussed below, and the circumstances in which they may be chosen for pain therapy are highlighted.

Intravenous route

The main advantage of the i.v. route is the rapid attainment of therapeutic blood levels, because the drug is introduced directly into the systemic circulation and bypasses the absorptive mechanisms and first-pass metabolism. It follows that any untoward effect will be similarly rapid in onset: this may include overwhelming anaphylaxis with any drug, or respiratory depression with intravenous opioids. Anyone using this route must be prepared to deal immediately and competently with any potentially life-threatening adverse effects.

The advantage of a rapid onset of action is matched by the disadvantage of a rapid offset, which is overcome by using an intravenous infusion, or an alternative route if chronic dosing is required.

Both bolus injections and continuous infusions have been employed to treat acute and chronic pain. Continuous infusions have been shown to produce stable therapeutic blood levels, avoiding the problems of drug peaks and troughs (Figure 2.3) When drug levels are below therapeutic level the patient will be in pain: when the drug level is within the therapeutic band pain will be controlled. It follows that bolus injections, like oral medication taken as required (PRN), should not be used to treat chronic pain. An additional problem is that tolerance seems to develop rapidly when opioids are given intermittently as separate i.v. injections. Intravenous administration requires highly skilled staff to insert and maintain intravenous lines, expensive equipment and, in the great majority of cases, hospital time and treatment.

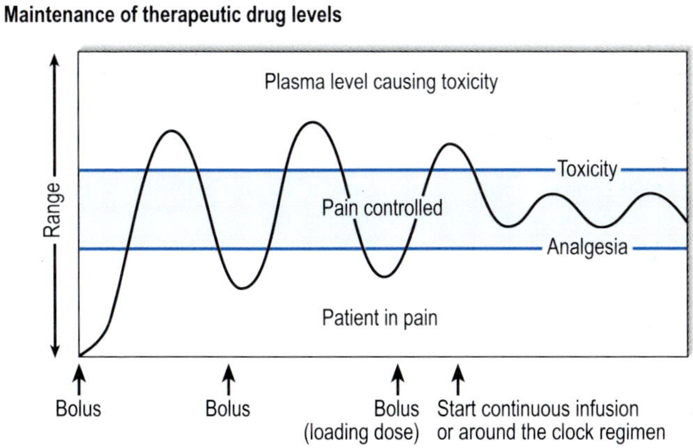

Fig. 2.3 Maintenance of therapeutic drug levels. N.B. The patient is intermittently in pain when the bolus regime is used. (Modified from Platt R 1993 Cancer pain. Lippincott-Raven, with permission.)

Uses of the intravenous route in pain management

- Intravenous therapy is indicated whenever an immediate response is vital, especially when there is hypovolaemia and therefore a poor peripheral circulation with unpredictable drug absorption, for example in the management of major trauma.
- Patient-controlled analgesia (PCA), a form of intravenous infusion, is commonly used in the management of postoperative pain. The patient may administer the drug intermittently only, or this option may be combined with a continuous background infusion.
- Continuous i.v. infusions of opioid are used in the management of cancer pain, although subcutaneous infusions are more usual.
- Intravenous analgesia is frequently used in intensive care units, postoperative recovery and high-dependency units.

Intramuscular injection

This technique, used since the late 19th century, is still the most common way of administering postoperative analgesia worldwide. It is not without hazard and has important disadvantages, but it is cheap, can be administered without complicated or expensive equipment, and the technique is quickly learned by a patient's relative or untrained carer.

The intramuscular (i.m.) route may be favoured when:

- analgesia is required and the patient is unable to take drugs by mouth
- compliance is in doubt
- when a rapid onset of effect is required but the intravenous route is impractical, for example in the management of the agitated or violent patient
- for prolonged duration of action: many hormones are given in this way: the contraceptive depoprovera is an example
- when oral administration is ineffective and other routes of administration are either contraindicated (as is the use of i.v. adrenaline in the treatment of anaphylaxis) or more hazardous than i.m. use.

The i.m. route has important drawbacks. There are complications associated with its use (see below) and, most importantly, absorption of a drug administered in this way is unpredictable, even for the same individual.

Absorption depends on:

- blood flow to the muscle: the greater the blood flow the better the absorption. For this reason the i.m. route is not suitable in the patient who is hypotensive or 'shut down'. Drug absorption will be poor while the patient is in this state, but if blood flow to the muscle improves the drug may then enter the circulation many hours later, when it may be hazardous
- the formulation of the drug. Some drugs, such as phenytoin, precipitate at the injection site, and this greatly reduces their absorption. A drug which is

poorly water soluble (lipophilicity is less important) will not be well absorbed as it must remain in solution at the injection site for absorption to occur. This is why diazepam should not be given by i.m. injection.

- the needle used for administering the drug. It has been shown that the depth of gluteal subcutaneous fat in both men over 70 kg and women is about 3.5 cm. Most injections are given by a 21-gauge needle, which has a total length of 3.8 cm, and of this 0.5 cm does not penetrate the skin. As blood flow to fat is minimal absorption will be very poor if too short a needle is used.

Local complications of the i.m. route

There is always some pain associated with an i.m. injection. The skin and subcutaneous tissues are densely innervated with pain receptors, which are stimulated by the needle passing through. The volume of the injectate is also important. A smaller volume will be less painful and there will be less distension of the interstitial space of the skeletal muscle. Some solutions are intrinsically irritating and therefore painful – sometimes local anaesthetics are mixed with such injectates and may reduce the pain.

Other local complications include:

- elevation of serum creatinine phosphokinase levels, which may cause diagnostic difficulties
- sciatic nerve damage is possible if the i.m. injection is made in the gluteal region
- haematoma formation: i.m. injections are contraindicated in fully anticoagulated patients, those on thrombolytic drugs or those with low platelet counts – **take care in haematology patients!**
- skin pigmentation and scarring
- cellulitis and local abscess formation
- sterile abscess formation, e.g. with diclofenac and paraldehyde
- very rarely, muscle fibrosis and contraction
- very rarely, tissue necrosis and gangrene.

There are possible systemic complications of i.m. injections but these are usually related to the drug itself rather than the route. An i.m. injection is more likely than an i.v. injection to be given by a practitioner with less training or outside a hospital setting: if the patient has an anaphylactic reaction the skills and equipment necessary to treat it may not be available.

Position of i.m. injections for analgesic drugs

- NSAIDS that can be given intramuscularly should be given in the gluteal muscles – the outer, upper quadrant of the buttock. Other positions are associated with local complications such as intense pain, skin necrosis and abscesses. **Do not give diclofenac i.m.**

- All other injections, except some vaccines, should be given into the vastus lateralis muscle (which has a thinner layer of subcutaneous fat) in the anterolateral part of the thigh. There is a much lower risk of nerve palsies with this position.

Intramuscular injections have a much higher complication rate in children. Be very careful.

Subcutaneous route

This is the introduction of drugs under the horny keratinous layer of the skin; it requires the use of a hypodermic needle. It may be chosen when the patient is unable to manage oral medication (because of nausea, vomiting or dysphagia, for example) and it is especially commonly used in the palliative care of cancer patients. Drugs may be given as separate boluses in the treatment of breakthrough or acute pain, but a continuous infusion is needed for chronic pain. Intermittent bolus therapy of opioids, for example, leads to peaks and troughs in drug levels – a cause of uneven pain relief ('the bolus effect') in association with drowsiness and emesis after each individual dose (See Figure 2.3).

The rate of absorption of a subcutaneous injection will depend on the local blood flow and the speed at which the drug diffuses away from the site of injection. Subcutaneous absorption of a drug tends to be faster than intramuscular, but it is unpredictable and this route should not be used when a rapid response is vital or when there is hypotension or hypovolaemia: blood flow to the skin will be reflexly reduced in these circumstances. The addition of hyaluronidase may speed up the absorption of a subcutaneously administered drug by breaking down the tissue matrix, and absorption will be increased when the ambient or body temperature increases. The addition of a vasoconstrictor such as adrenaline will reduce local blood flow to the skin and so reduce absorption. This is exploited to prolong the action of local anaesthetics and to reduce blood loss, but never to parts of the body with a single blood supply, such as a finger or toe (see Chapter 4).

Indications for use of the subcutaneous route

- Patient unable to take oral medication: it is especially useful in palliative care, where it is routine to give opioids, and other drugs, by a subcutaneous infusion pump, sometimes for weeks or months. Subcutaneous pumps can be used in the community. The European Working Party (1996) on morphine has stated that it is the preferred alternative route when oral medication can no longer be used.
- Patient-controlled analgesia is sometimes administered subcutaneously.

Some drugs are too irritant to be used by the subcutaneous route, for example pethidine and prochlorperazine.

Rectal route

The mechanism of drug absorption from the rectum is very similar to that from the upper GI tract (i.e. passive diffusion), but the surface area available in the rectum (200–400 cm^2) is much smaller than that of the small intestine (about 2 000 000 cm^2).

The rectal route can be used:

- if the patient is unconscious, unable to swallow or nil by mouth for any reason
- when a patient has nausea or vomiting
- for a direct effect on the rectum and proximal large bowel, for example in the treatment of constipation
- if the drug has a foul taste (this may be useful in children)
- if the patient is being nursed at home and relatives or untrained attendants need to give drugs
- in emergencies, as some of a drug in solution will pass directly into the systemic circulation. An example is the control of fitting with rectal diazepam
- where financial constraints limit the availability of the trained staff and equipment needed to give subcutaneous infusions.

Although drugs in alkaline aqueous solution will be rapidly absorbed this is not a practical option for anything except short-term use. The rate-limiting step in absorption from a suppository is the transport of drug from the fatty vehicle to the rectal fluid. Small differences in manufacturers' formulations can lead to large differences in absorption rates.

The rectum has a good blood supply and venous drainage takes place into both the portal (mostly the upper part of the rectum) and the systemic circulations (the lower part of the rectum). Venous anastomoses exist but their extent varies between different individuals, so an unpredictable proportion of an absorbed drug will pass directly into the systemic circulation, bypassing presystemic metabolism. A suppository placed low in the rectum, in contact with the mucosa, will be likely to deliver its drug directly into the systemic circulation. Therefore a high-clearance drug, e.g. morphine, may have a greater than expected pharmacological effect from a given dose and individual titration will be especially important. Once a dose is established for a patient the absorption tends to remain consistent unless a new problem, such as constipation, arises. An advantage of the rectal route is that in the event of an overdose or adverse effect the remainder of the preparation can be easily removed.

Important disadvantages of the rectal route include:

- A full rectum will hinder the absorption of the drug. This may be pertinent in the management of cancer pain with opioids, as these drugs cause constipation.
- Drugs are absorbed too slowly in suppository form for it to be used in the treatment of acute pain, or when a rapid onset of action is needed.
- The small surface area of the rectum may delay or limit absorption.
- There is only a small quantity of rectal fluid (3–4 ml), so the dissolution of any drug vehicle, to allow drug absorption, may be slow.
- Suppositories may be extruded from the rectum before absorption of the drug, and defecation may be triggered by the insertion of an irritant drug.
- Rectal irritation may occur with prolonged continuous use of this route.
- With normal release morphine, for example, 3–4-hourly insertion of suppositories will be necessary to maintain analgesia.
- Patients may dislike the idea of rectal drugs.
- An elderly or frail individual may not be able to self-medicate.
- A painful rectal condition, e.g. an anal fissure, would make the use of this route impossible.

In summary, the rectal route can be used to obtain local and systemic therapeutic effects. It has been less frequently employed in the management of cancer pain in the western world since the introduction of syringe drivers, but its simplicity and cheapness make it a useful option if careful attention is paid to dose titration.

Transdermal administration

The intact skin provides a protective barrier to retain water and other bodily fluids and to keep out infection and injurious substances. This barrier is not impenetrable. It has long been observed that the systemic side-effects of steroid therapy could develop after topical application.

In recent years a number of transdermal patch formulations have been developed to allow the delivery of drugs across the skin. In pain therapy transdermal delivery is used to achieve both local anaesthesia (EMLA cream) and systemic pain relief (fentanyl, for example). A drug which is to have a systemic effect needs to be absorbed through the skin into the systemic circulation.

Transdermal delivery for systemic effects

The intact stratum corneum, or outer horny layer, provides the rate-limiting step to the percutaneous absorption of drugs through the skin. In fact, low molecular weight lipophilic substances will be absorbed slowly into this layer, which will then provide a reservoir for the slow release of drugs. Only a

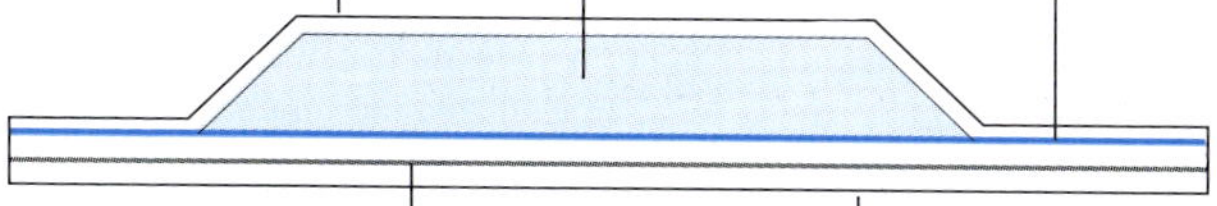

Fig. 2.4 Schematic (cross-sectional) representation of fentanyl patch (After Janssen-Cilag.).

small amount of a potent substance is needed to produce a pharmacological effect (this can be seen when an atopic individual is exposed to a small amount of foreign protein to which he is allergic – anaphylaxis may result). Substances which are only hydrophilic will be very poorly absorbed.

A diagrammatic representation of a transdermal patch is shown in Figure 2.4, where fentanyl is used as an example. In some transdermal delivery systems a large amount of drug is released immediately as soon as the patch makes contact with the skin. This initial bolus quickly raises plasma levels of the drug to the therapeutic range, and then a continuous amount is released steadily over the lifetime of the patch.

Fentanyl. Reaches analgesic concentrations within 6–12 hours (there is considerable interindividual variation). Levels continue to rise for 12–18 hours, plasma levels then remain constant for the next 72 hours, when a new patch is needed. There will be a reservoir of drug in the stratum corneum, which will continue to be released in the first 12–18 hours after removal of a patch.

The reservoir of drug remaining in the skin should always be remembered: deaths have occurred when transdermal fentanyl has been used to treat acute pain. As the painful stimulus recedes, even if the patch is removed the drug will continue to leach into the systemic circulation and respiratory depression will result.

Another way in which the problems of transdermal drug delivery have been partially overcome is shown by EMLA cream. High drug concentrations are needed to penetrate the stratum corneum with any success, and most topical emulsions have about 20% in the base form. EMLA contains a eutectic mixture of lignocaine and prilocaine, i.e. the combination has a lower melting point than either of the two constituent drugs. Above 16°C it exists as an oil with a very high concentration of the two anaesthetics in the droplets. It is most commonly used to provide local anaesthesia for venepuncture in children. Amethocaine gel (see Chapter 4) is a newer alternative to EMLA.

Other factors which affect drug release include the regional differences in the thickness of the stratum corneum and its degree of hydration. Penetration of drugs may be 10 times greater on the face than on the trunk, and drug absorption is much greater in well hydrated skin. Transdermal patches increase drug absorption by acting as occlusive dressings, trapping moisture in the horny layer. Increased body temperature will also increase drug absorption: local skin temperature is raised by the transdermal device.

Unwanted effects of transdermal drugs include local skin irritation, which may prevent continued use as it can only be treated by removal of the patch. Successive patches should always be put in a different place in the same anatomical region to reduce the incidence of this problem. Unwanted systemic effects of the drug must also be remembered.

Buccal and sublingual route

Buccal means the medicine is placed between the upper lip and the lining of the upper gum. A sublingual drug is placed under the tongue.

Drugs absorbed from the mouth, rather than swallowed, pass directly into the systemic circulation and bypass first-pass metabolism. If they have the right physicochemical properties (being very fat-soluble is most important) absorption is very rapid, as the mouth is richly supplied with blood vessels and lymphatics.

The sublingual route is important in pain relief to:

- bypass first-pass metabolism: although several opioids undergo appreciable first-pass metabolism only buprenorphine and phenazocine are given by this route routinely
- allow rapid absorption: for example, dextromoramide is sometimes used by this route as a rapidly acting analgesic for breakthrough pain
- allow treatment of local conditions such as mouth ulcers with local anaesthetics.

The buccal route has been used in dying patients when the subcutaneous or other parenteral routes could not be used, as a tablet under the upper or lower lip will not easily be dislodged and will permit analgesia to be given by family or other untrained carers and with minimal equipment. The Expert Working Group of the European Association for Palliative Care has recommended that the buccal and sublingual routes be **avoided** in cancer pain therapy, as they have no clinical advantages over conventional routes and drug absorption is unpredictable.

Spinal analgesia

The discovery of endogenous opioid receptors and ligands in the brain and spinal cord, and the observation of analgesic activity of intrathecal opioids in rats, led to the idea of placing opioid analgesics intraspinally to effect pain relief in patients. There are a large number of both opioid and non-opioid receptors in the spinal cord which are involved in the modulation of pain signals, some to reduce and some to augment nociception. The dorsal horns contain the most dense concentration of opioid receptors (in Rexed laminae II and III, the substantia gelatinosa). They are present both pre- and postsynaptically and, as elsewhere, have an inhibitory effect on the transmission of pain. The action of intraspinal opioids is not confined to the spinal cord: cephalad migration of opioids in the CSF means that brain opioid receptors are involved in analgesia, and systemic absorption of opioids also takes place. It follows that systemic unwanted effects of opioids will also occur.

It is important to remember that intraspinal analgesia potentially has a much greater morbidity, and mortality, than any other administration route. The complication rate is related to the experience of the practitioner, but in any hands it is more hazardous for the patient. It should only be used when there are well-founded reasons for choosing it above simpler methods of pain relief. The risk – benefit ratio for the individual patient is crucial in the decision to choose it.

The term intraspinal includes both epidural and intrathecal injection, and both routes will be discussed together in this section, but the important differences between them must first be highlighted. Intrathecal medication is deposited in the subarachnoid space and epidural drugs are placed in the epidural space (Figure 2.5).

The intraspinal route has been used in:

- the management of postoperative pain, especially post-thoracotomy and major abdominal surgery
- the management of pain in labour, for operative delivery and prenatal surgical procedures
- for pain relief during surgery, both as part of a mixed technique with general anaesthesia and as sole method of analgesia
- the management of pain relief in trauma
- the management of chronic non-malignant pain
- the management of cancer pain.

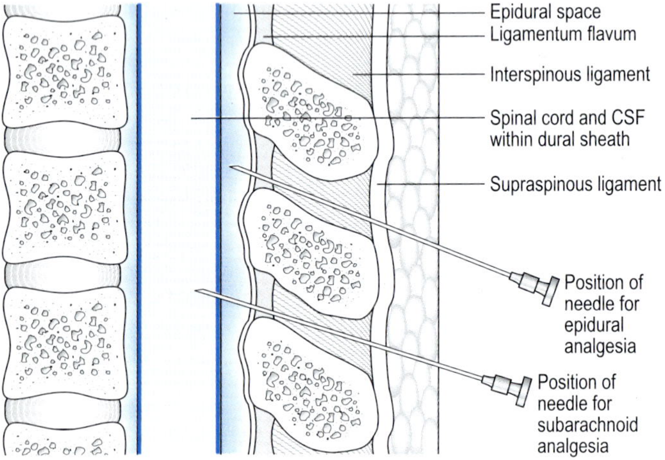

Fig. 2.5 Placement of epidural drugs in the epidural space and intrathecal drugs in the subarachnoid space.

Unwanted effects from the intraspinal route

Neurological damage. This has occurred from the administration of many sorts of solution, both accidentally (total parenteral nutrition solution, thiopentone, pancuronium) and deliberately (when an established drug has been tried by this new route). This complication can only be prevented by highly trained staff using safe techniques, for example two members of staff checking any drug (and the dose) which is to be given intraspinally and labelling infusion lines clearly.

Most instances of misplaced drugs or solutions have resulted in self-limiting back pain and spasm, but paraplegia has been reported (e.g. with vinca alkaloids). Treatments that have been used on these occasions include trying to withdraw the drug back through the catheter or syringe, dilution with saline and the administration of epidural steroids.

Systemic effects. Drugs administered intraspinally will also be taken up systemically: the epidural space contains large numbers of blood vessels and plasma concentrations of opioids are almost equal to those that follow intravenous and intramuscular administration. All the adverse effects of systemic opioids should be expected and treated. These include:

- nausea and vomiting
- sedation
- constipation.

The unwanted effects of local anaesthetics and other drugs should be anticipated and treated.

Pruritus. This is very common after intrathecal opioids, particularly in opioid-naive patients. Antihistamines have been used but with mixed success.

Urinary symptoms. Urinary retention after intraspinally administered opioids is well documented: it is due to decreased detrusor muscle tone and detrusor–urethral sphincter incoordination.

Infections. Infections can occur anywhere from the skin to the meninges. Serious infection (meningitis or epidural abscess) has not emerged as a common complication of intraspinal drug therapy.

Infection may occur:

- at the catheter exit site
- along the deep or superficial catheter track
- in the epidural or subarachnoid space.

If undetected and untreated, deep infection can have serious neurological sequelae from meningitis or the formation of an epidural abscess, with vascular compromise and permanent neurological damage.

Superficial infections can be detected by sight through clear dressings and the patient may complain of soreness. Treatment with systemic antibiotics should resolve the problem.

Epidural space infections are associated with constant, non-specific back pain, pain on injection, oedema near the proximal incision and reduced analgesia. Meningism and fever or neurological abnormalities are rare.

Infections should first be avoided by meticulous attention to aseptic technique, good skin care and vigilance after the insertion of the catheter. Patients should be instructed in what to look for and to report back to the unit if the signs or symptoms of problems develop. Carers in the community should also be told the danger signs. If infection is suspected vigorous early treatment, including removal of the catheter, is indicated.

The source of infections in a recent series included:

- the skin
- the injectate
- bloodborne spread from sites of infection elsewhere in the patient.

Systemic infection, or a site of infection near to the planned insertion of an intraspinal injection, is normally a contraindication to the technique unless an experienced clinician and the patient have decided the risk is outweighed by potential benefits.

Spinal headache. In a subarachnoid injection the meninges are broached and there is leakage of CSF: this is associated with a spinal headache. It is thought that the inequality in pressure which results from this leakage causes traction on the meninges, resulting in a severe frontal headache which is relieved only when the patient lies flat. The headache may last a week or more. Simple analgesics may also help and if the headache is severe the hole can be closed by the anaesthetist inserting a 'blood patch'. This involves finding the epidural space, by the usual aseptic method, and injecting some of the patient's venous blood into it.

The severity of the headache is related to:

- size of needle: an epidural needle (usually 14 or 16 G) accidentally inserted into the arachnoid mater will cause a large hole and greater CSF leakage, with a greater likelihood of headache. Small spinal needles (up to 29 G have been used) are associated with a much smaller risk
- patient characteristics: even with small spinal needles the risk of headache is much greater in obstetric practice; the elderly seem to suffer it less frequently even with certain CSF leakage.

The risks and benefits of intraspinal analgesia should be carefully weighed in patients with:

- clotting abnormalities: a bleeding diathesis increases the risk of epidural haematoma, with consequent pressure on nerve roots and neurological damage. Patients fully anticoagulated on warfarin or heparin should not have intraspinal analgesia, although low-dose aspirin (75 mg) has not been associated with problems. Clotting studies should be done in cases of doubt
- septicaemia: there is a risk of introducing infection into the CNS
- diabetes: patients on insulin are at greater risk of infection.

NB: The patient who is receiving continuing intraspinal analgesia needs specialized care – its absence may make this technique unsuitable.

Intrathecal route

This is the deposition of drugs into the subarachnoid space under the arachnoid mater.

Epidural route (Table 2.3)

The epidural space is a potential space which extends from the sacral hiatus to the base of the skull, and lies within the vertebral canal between the dura mater and the ligamentum flavum. This route provides indirect access to central pain receptors, the site of action being identical to that of drugs delivered intrathecally, i.e. the spinal roots, mixed spinal nerves and the surface of the spinal cord to a depth of about 1 mm. In a successful epidural injection the meninges are not broached, so that headache from CSF leakage should not be a problem and the risk of meningitis is minimized.

TABLE 2.3 Potential advantages of epidural and intrathecal placement (modified from Platt R 1993 Cancer Pain. Lippincott–Raven, with permission)

Epidural placement	*Intrathecal placement*
Meninges not broached, therefore reduced risk of spinal headache	Technically easier to locate the subarachnoid space
Lower risk of meningitis as dura intact – infection risk limited to epidural abscess	Less risk of catheter obstruction by epidural fibrosis or metastases
Greater flexibility in choice of drugs used – lipophilic agents and local anaesthetics can be used safely and effectively	Less painful on insertion
Unwanted effects less common and less extreme	Analgesia more rapid in onset and more complete
Greater flexibility in site selection – rostral placement may be combined with a lipophilic opioid for more segmental analgesia	Lower doses and volume of opioid are required to produce analgesia (about 1/10 the systemic dose of morphine, for example)
Risk of neurological injury smaller	The risk of catheter migration is minimal
Margin of safety increased in case of accidental overdose	

Inhalational route

Drugs may be inhaled through the mouth or the nose: they will then be absorbed into the rich blood supply of the lungs and thence into the systemic circulation. Drugs are given by this route both for local and systemic effects.

When a drug is nebulized an aerosol is produced. An aerosol is a physical system in which particles are dispersed in a gas. The drug in liquid form, for example morphine in solution, is deposited in the reservoir of the nebulizer and air or oxygen is piped through it. Liquid particles are generated by this method, varying in size from about 2 to 20 μm across. Only the smallest particles – less than 5 μm – will reach the bronchioles and alveoli. The larger particles will be deposited in the upper airways and be absorbed into the systemic circulation. Some drug-containing particles are trapped in the mucus and cleared by mucociliary action. Only 10–20% of an administered dose reaches the lungs. Only 5% of a given dose of nebulized morphine, for example, will reach the systemic circulation. There is no evidence to suggest that morphine exerts its effect through local opioid receptors, and it is the absorbed proportion that is pharmacologically active.

Although nebulized drugs are commonly used in other branches of medicine there are not enough controlled data or clinical experience to make recommendations about the use of inhaled analgesics in routine pain management practice.

The most common form of inhaled pain relief is the gas Entonox (see Chapter 13 for more details).

CHAPTER 3

THE OPIOIDS

MORPHINE

This is the standard 'strong' opioid and a powerful μ agonist. It is the drug of first choice in the treatment of severe nociceptive pain. Some of its pain-relieving properties are thought to be mediated by an active metabolite, morphine-6-glucuronide (M6G). Morphine is the main pharmacologically active constituent of opium, which is extracted from the poppy *Papaver somniferum*.

PHARMACOKINETICS

Morphine administration can be oral, rectal, subcutaneous, intramuscular, intravenous and intraspinal.

Oral absorption

Morphine is well absorbed from the GI tract, mostly in the proximal small bowel. First-pass metabolism is extensive, so that although oral absorption is good oral bioavailability is generally stated to be approximately 25% (a range of 15–64% has been reported).

The plasma half-life of morphine is 3 hours. The plasma half-life of M6G is slightly over 3 hours in healthy people, and markedly increased in renal failure.

Peak analgesia

Peak analgesia occurs:

- within 30–60 minutes of oral administration of an ordinary release preparation
- within 2–4 hours of administration of an oral modified-release preparation, depending on the one chosen
- within 30–60 minutes of rectal administration
- 20–60 minutes after subcutaneous (s.c.) administration
- 20–60 minutes after intramuscular (i.m.) administration
- 5–20 minutes after an intravenous (i.v.) injection
- 30 minutes after lumbar intrathecal (i.t.) injection.

Analgesia lasts 4–6 hours.

Metabolism

This takes place principally in the liver, and glucuronidation and oxidation are the principal reactions. The main metabolites are morphine-3-glucuronide (M3G) and morphine-6-glucuronide (M6G). In liver disease morphine metabolism is not affected until liver function is severely impaired. Extrahepatic sites of morphine metabolism include the CNS but not the kidney in healthy individuals.

The pharmacological actions of M6G are identical to those of morphine, but M6G has twice the analgesic potency: in animal studies, when it has been given intracerebrally the potency is 100 times that of morphine. It is likely that M6G is responsible for a very significant portion of the analgesic effects of morphine in **chronic** use, and may account for the different oral to parenteral dose ratios of morphine in chronic (1:3) and single-dose studies (1:6). In renal failure M6G accumulates, which helps explain the longer half-life and duration of analgesia in patients with this condition.

Morphine-induced pain ('paradoxical pain')

There have been reports that when morphine is used at very high doses intrathecally or intravenously the patient's pain may actually increase. Most of the cases reported so far have been in patients with cancer. One hypothetical explanation for this phenomenon is that abnormal metabolism of morphine may occur, so that relatively greater quantities of the antagonistic metabolite M3G are produced relative to the analgesic M6G.

Renal impairment and the excretion of morphine

The metabolism of morphine is not impaired in renal failure but the **excretion** of morphine, and its principal metabolites, is. The accumulation of M6G can cause respiratory depression. It is especially important to **titrate the dose of morphine against the pain** in these patients.

THERAPEUTIC USES IN PAIN RELIEF

- Severe nociceptive pain – for example cancer pain.
- Severe acute pain – for example postoperative pain.
- Neuropathic pain – this may be opioid poorly responsive; more rarely it is non-responsive.

Unwanted effects

These are common to all opioids but the incidence and severity vary with different drugs, so that if a patient cannot tolerate one opioid after active management of the unwanted effect, another of comparable efficacy should be tried, e.g. substituting methadone for morphine in the management of cancer pain. Table 3.1 shows the management of the unwanted effects of opioids.

TABLE 3.1 Management of the unwanted effects of morphine

Symptom	*Causes*	*Management*
Respiratory depression	Direct effect on μ receptors in the pons and medulla: rate, depth and rhythm of respiration altered, leading to CO_2 retention	**Titrate dose against pain.** i.v./s.c. naloxone + artificial ventilation may be necessary
Nausea and vomiting	Due to stimulation of chemoreceptor trigger zone (central effect) and gastric stasis (peripheral effect)	Antiemetics: haloperidol 1.5–3 mg b.d. s.c. p.o. (CTZ) or metoclopramide 10–20 mg t.d.s.
Constipation	Direct effect on smooth muscle of GI tract	Regular dose of stimulant + softening laxative. Great range in dose needed for control of constipation
Sedation	Central effect of morphine	Reduce dose of morphine if feasible, titrate dose against the pain, consider trial of psychostimulant (e.g. dexamphetamine or methylphenidate) if all else fails
Movement-related nausea and vomiting	Vestibular stimulation	Cyclizine 50–100 mg p.o./s.c.
Urinary retention	Increased smooth muscle tone in urinary tract	Catherization may be necessary
Pruritus	Histamine release in the skin	Oral antihistamine
Bronchoconstriction	Histamine release in the bronchial tree	i.v./i.m. antihistamine with a bronchodilator **Change to another opioid** immediately
Psychomimetic effects	Dysphoria, hallucinations and nightmares	Haloperidol 3–5 mg p.o./s.c. nocte
Morphine-induced pain: with **high dose i.v. and i.t.** administration	Accumulation of M3G, which is an antagonist of the analgesic effects of morphine	May need to switch to alternative opioid, e.g. methadone, for severe pain

Contraindications to the use of morphine

The use of morphine is contraindicated in the following cases:

- Patients with raised intracranial pressure (including all those with a significant head injury) because, when spontaneously breathing, the respiratory depressant effect may cause an increase in arterial PCO_2 and intracranial pressure will rise still further
- Patients with biliary colic: an NSAID or pethidine is preferred by some surgeons, as morphine is said to raise muscle tone, and therefore pressure, in the biliary tract. There is no evidence to support this widely taught belief.
- Patients with aspirin-sensitive asthma may be more likely to suffer an allergic reaction to those morphine preparations that contain sulphites.

Precautions in the use of morphine

Morphine and the neonate

Neonates feel pain and may require morphine perioperatively. The plasma half-life is significantly longer and there is greater respiratory depression for an equivalent adult dose, as morphine crosses the immature blood–brain barrier more easily. In babies born at term, morphine clearance reaches adult levels by the age of 1 month.

Morphine and children

Healthy children are no more sensitive to morphine than adults, but the dose should be **titrated against the pain**.

Morphine in old age

Morphine requirements fall with age: this is related to the decrease in creatinine clearance that is a normal part of ageing. It may be necessary to decrease both the size and number of daily doses of morphine that are given.

Obstetric patients

Morphine is not favoured in obstetric patients. There is some evidence that it delays the onset of established labour when used in stage I. Use in the mother may also cause respiratory depression in the newborn child, as it will cross the immature blood–brain barrier more easily.

Lactating mothers

Only small amounts of morphine are excreted into breast milk, so the usual therapeutic doses for the mother should not affect the infant. In a mother who is a drug abuser using diamorphine, the higher doses needed for her may cause respiratory depression in a baby who is being breastfed. Babies born to addicted mothers will also be at risk of opioid withdrawal syndrome.

ADMINISTRATION

Oral morphine

This is the route of choice in chronic use (e.g. for cancer pain). It is effective, non-invasive and allows the patient greater independence. It is also cheaper.

Morphine is now available in many forms, both normal release (4-hourly administration) and modified release (once and twice daily) as solutions, tablets and granules.

> **Parenteral morphine has no greater efficacy than oral morphine, but may be needed, even in chronic pain, when the patient cannot take drugs by mouth.**

Starting dose of oral morphine

This depends on the patient's age, general condition and previous medication. Whether the patient is in hospital or at home will also influence the choice. A frail elderly patient, or one with serious hepatic or respiratory problems, should be started on a dose which is likely to be too small rather than too large; the dose can then be titrated upwards to achieve the best possible pain control.

Converting to oral morphine (more detail is given in 'Clinical use of morphine', Chapter 14)

- Add up the usual dose of opioid used in a 24-hour period, in milligrams.
- Multiply this by the **relative potency** of the opioid in question. This will give the total daily dose of morphine that will give approximately equivalent relief.
- If pain control has been unsatisfactory then the total daily dose of morphine should be increased by about 50%.
- If using normal-release tablets or solution, divide the total by 6 to give the 4-hourly starting dose. It may need to be rounded to the nearest 5 or 10 mg.
- If using modified-release (m/r) release morphine, divide by 2 and round up to the nearest convenient twice-daily dose.

Rectal morphine

This route is little used for adults in the UK because the subcutaneous route is generally preferred for patients unable to swallow. It may occasionally be useful, especially in the community, if oral administration is not practicable and there is to be a delay before a subcutaneous infusion can be started. It is also easier to teach an untrained carer to insert a suppository than give an injection.

> **It is not advisable to give modified-release preparations per rectum, per vaginam or into a colostomy, as absorption is unpredictable.**

Parenteral morphine

Intravenous use

Anyone giving bolus doses of morphine or other opioids must be prepared and equipped to treat apnoea and have resuscitation equipment, such as an ambubag, oxygen and naloxone, available. The unwanted effects of morphine are more likely when the drug is administered rapidly intravenously, and it is far better to give small increments, observing for the desired effect, than to treat adverse effects. A suggested rate of administration for an adult is 2 mg/min, but the patient's previous exposure to opioids and response to them will be the best guide.

Subcutaneous morphine

This route is commonly used in palliative care, where subcutaneous infusions of opioids and other drugs are sometimes used for some months for ambulant patients at home who cannot take oral medication. It is also used to give as required (PRN) for 'breakthrough pain.'

Intramuscular morphine

This is a common route for morphine administration in the acute setting. Doses are usually calculated for the patient's weight, i.e. a normal adult will require 0.2 mg/kg, but this can only be a guide and it is important to **titrate the dose against the pain**.

Intrathecal and epidural morphine (Table 3.2)

This is the placement of morphine into either the subarachnoid space (intrathecal, i.t.) or the epidural space (e.d.). Both of these techniques are

Table 3.2 The specific advantages of intrathecal and epidural opioids

Intrathecal	*Epidural*
Much lower dose of opioid needed than when used systematically	Lower dose of morphine needed than when used systematically
Regional specificity possible	No motor/autonomic effects
No motor/autonomic effects	Lower incidence of adverse effects than i.t. use (neurotoxicity, meningitis)
Longer duration of action than other routes	Longer duration of action than other routes
Availability of specific antagonist – naloxone	Availability of specific antagonist – naloxone

invasive and should only be used if there is a specific indication (see Chapter 2), or if simpler methods have failed.

Respiratory depression from intraspinal opioids

The main disadvantage of i.t. and e.d. administration, apart from those always associated with these routes, is the possibility of respiratory depression. This has been reported **up to 24 hours** after the use of epidural morphine in opioid-naive postoperative patients, when it is called 'late respiratory depression'. Both early and late respiratory depression occur with intrathecal opioids.

Risk factors for respiratory depression include:

- opioid naivete: late respiratory depression has been reported in patients given intraspinal opioids for postoperative pain. These people had not received opioids before. It has not been reported in cancer patients on long-term opioid therapy, who are treated with intrathecal morphine
- overdose of opioid
- absence of severe pain: in the treatment of acute postoperative pain, when the painful stimulus decreases if the dose of opioid is not reduced the patient is at risk of respiratory depression. Since the dose must be titrated against the pain a simpler, more flexible analgesic method may be more appropriate
- simultaneous administration of opioids by other routes
- advanced age
- frailty
- coexisting respiratory disease
- sleep apnoea
- simultaneous administration of other CNS depressants.

The respiratory depression that can follow intraspinal opioids is sometimes very sudden, and may not be preceded by a progressive fall in respiratory rate or level of consciousness.

Buccal and sublingual morphine

Tablets may be placed between the lining of the upper lip and the gum above the upper front teeth – this is buccal administration. The subcutaneous route is more usual now. Sublingual administration is not commonly used for morphine.

Transdermal morphine

This is not currently used for morphine but iontophoresis may make it a possibility in the future.

The pharmacological properties of other opioids are summarized in Table 3.3. Important differences between morphine and commonly used opioids are outlined below.

TABLE 3.3 Pharmacological characteristics of some common opioids

Opioid	*Receptor activity*	*Routes of administration*	*Relative potency to morphine p.o.*	*O:P ratio*	*Onset (min)*	*Peak (min)*	*$T^1/_2$ (h)*	*Duration of pain relief (h)*
Fentanyl	μ agonist	i.v. transdermal, e.d.	n/a	n/a	5 i.v.		2 i.v.	0.4–0.5 i.v.
Phenazocine	μ agonist	s.l., o	5.0	1:0.4	20	45–60	?	6
Diamorphine	μ agonist	o, i.v., s.c., i.m., e.d.	1.5	1:2.5	20–30	30–45	3	4–6
Oxycodone	μ agonist	o, p.r., i.v., i.m.	1.3 p.o. 0.75 i.m.	1:2	15–30		4–5	4
Methadone	μ agonist	o, s.c., i.m. p.r., buccal	1.0 single 3–4 repeated	1:2	30–60	30–120	15 8–80	6–8
Nalbuphine	Mixed agonist/ antagonist	i.m., s.c., i.v.	1.0	1:4–1:5	15–30	45–60	5	5–6
Morphine	μ agonist	o, i.v., s.c., i.m., p.r. i.t., e.d.	1.0	1:3	30–60	60–90	3	4–6
Papaveretum	μ agonist	i.m., o	0.5–0.75	1:3	60	60–90	3	4
Tramadol	μ, δ, κ agonism + non-opioid	o, p.r., i.v., i.m., s.c.	0.25	1:4	20–60	30–60	4–6	6
Pethidine	μ agonist	o, s.c., i.m., i.v.	0.125	1:3	30–60	60–120	2.5	2–4
Meptazinol	Partial μ agonist + central cholinergic properties	p.o., i.m.	?	1:2	?	?	2–4	2 (3–5 in elderly)
Dextropropoxyphene	Weak μ agonist	o	0.16	N/A	30	60–120	12	4–6
Dihydrocodeine	Weak μ agonist	o, i.m.	0.1	1:3	30	45–60	3	4
Codeine	Prodrug	o, i.m.	0.1	1:1.5	30	45–60	3	4
Pentazocine	Mixed agonist/ antagonist	o, s.c., i.v., i.m.	0.06	1:4	40–60	60–180	2	2–4

DIAMORPHINE (DIACETYLMORPHINE, HEROIN)

This is a semisynthetic morphine analogue. It is a prodrug, rapidly converted in the body to morphine, monoacetylmorphine and M6G. The UK and Canada are the only two countries where it is available for medicinal purposes.

Oral absorption is rapid, but first-pass metabolism is almost complete. Although many authorities quote a conversion of 1.5 morphine to 1.0 diamorphine when changing drugs for oral administration, it is considered safe to use a 1:1 ratio (diamorphine to morphine) for chronic therapy and always to **titrate the dose against the pain**, as the conversion ratio for an individual patient may be very different. When changing from oral morphine to oral diamorphine some authorities advise using a ratio of 2:1.

Diamorphine has a more rapid onset of action than morphine and produces euphoria when used intravenously. The only clinical advantage that diamorphine has over morphine is its greater solubility, so that a much smaller volume is used parenterally. It remains the strong opioid of choice for subcutaneous use in the UK.

CODEINE

This is the parent drug of step 2 of the WHO Analgesic Pain Ladder (see Chapter 2), but it is rarely used as a sole analgesic in the UK because of a high incidence of unwanted effects – primarily nausea and constipation – so that there is a ceiling (see Chapter 2) to its analgesia. It is a prodrug which is converted to morphine in the body. This metabolic pathway is subject to genetic polymorphism, and 10% of the population are unable to make the conversion.

Compound analgesics contain both an opioid and a non-opioid (Table 3.4). The opioid may be present in low or normal dose. The low-dose opioid compounds may still cause opioid-related adverse effects, especially in the elderly. The disadvantages of fixed-dose compounds in general is that they do not offer flexibility: both components of the drug must be increased at the same time. Compound analgesics are, however, useful in pain management: coproxamol is the standard step 2 analgesic for many hospices in the UK, as it is efficacious and better tolerated than codeine in most patients. Coproxamol is more potent when used regularly than in single doses, because of the accumulation of dextropropoxyphene, which has a long half-life of 12–15 hours. Two tablets of coproxamol taken every 6 hours is equivalent to 6 mg of oral morphine regularly, and a patient will require 10 mg of morphine 4-hourly as a starting dose when switching drugs because of inadequate pain control.

TABLE 3.4 The formulation of some common compound analgesics

Drug name	*Contains*	*Notes on use*
Coproxamol	32.5 mg dextropropoxyphene 325 mg paracetamol	Very hazardous in overdose (opioid + paracetamol) Avoid in those on warfarin Inhibits carbamezepine metabolism Avoid in renal impairment (opioid accumulates)
Tylex	Codeine phosphate 30 mg Paracetamol 500 mg	Significant sodium content Avoid in renal impairment
Solpadol	Codeine phosphate 30 mg Paracetamol 500 mg	Avoid in renal impairment Has significant Na^+ content
Cocodamol	Codeine phosphate 8 mg Paracetamol 500 mg	Note low dose of opioid
Codydramol	Dihydrocodeine tartrate 10 mg Paracetamol 500 mg	Note low dose of opioid

PETHIDINE (MEPERIDINE IN THE USA)

This is a synthetic opioid analgesic which has μ agonist properties and anticholinergic effects. It is not suitable for use in chronic pain relief because of the accumulation of a toxic metabolite, norpethidine. Pethidine has antitussive effects only when used in analgesic doses; it is less constipating than morphine and more emetic. Many clinicians believe it causes less smooth muscle spasm than morphine (there is no evidence to support this); other differences are discussed below.

Many authorities believe that the use of pethidine should be avoided, as it offers no advantages over other opioids and carries the risk of significant toxicity.

PHARMACOKINETICS

Pethidine is well absorbed by all routes of administration, but as there is extensive hepatic first-pass metabolism oral administration is unreliable. Its oral to parenteral ratio is about 3:1. In patients with significant hepatic impairment oral bioavailability is greatly increased, from 50% to about 90%.

The **plasma half-life is 2–2.5 hours** and the **duration of analgesia about 2–4 hours**: it is often prescribed 4–6 hourly, which leads to poor pain control.

Pethidine is an irritant solution and should not be used by the subcutaneous route.

Metabolism

This takes place mainly in the liver. Norpethidine is an important metabolite because it is pharmacologically active and has a substantially longer half-life (8–21 hours) than pethidine itself. Norpethidine has only half the analgesic activity of its parent, but is a potent CNS stimulant – its accumulation leads to irritability and nervousness, tremors, myoclonic jerks, twitches and eventually convulsions.

Norpethidine accumulation is more likely to occur:

- with chronic high dosing of the drug
- in renal and hepatic impairment, when the half-life may be prolonged to more than 30 hours.

THERAPEUTIC USES IN PAIN MANAGEMENT

Pethidine is used in the relief of moderate to severe nociceptive pain. It is favoured in obstetric practice as it is reputed to cause less neonatal respiratory depression than morphine, but there is no evidence to support this. Its use in biliary and renal colic is being superseded by NSAIDs.

Precautions and contraindications

Pethidine should not be used for chronic pain relief (e.g. cancer pain) or in other situations where there is a danger of norpethidine accumulation (e.g. renal or hepatic impairment).

Pethidine is contraindicated in patients who have received monoamine oxidase inhibitors (MAOI) in the previous 14 days. The interaction between these drugs is thought to produce an accumulation of serotonin, and within minutes of the administration of pethidine the patient may become restless and violent, and may then develop fatal respiratory depression, severe hypertension and dysrhythmias.

Pethidine also has some vagolytic activity. It should therefore be used with caution in patients with supraventricular tachycardias or acute myocardial disease.

FENTANYL

Fentanyl citrate is well established as an intravenous μ agonist for perioperative use, its low incidence of histamine release making it especially suitable for patients with cardiovascular disease and atopy. It is structurally related to pethidine. More recently (1994) it has been produced in a transdermal form (TTS-fentanyl), which is finding a place in cancer pain management. More experience, and randomized controlled trials, will be needed before the clear indications for TTS-fentanyl are known.

Fentanyl cannot be given orally but it has a very rapid onset of action by the i.v. route. The short duration of analgesia is due to its rapid redistribution, as it is a very lipophilic drug. It is also given by the e.d. route in obstetric practice. The plasma half-life is 2 hours.

Peak analgesia occurs:

- within 2–3 minutes of an intravenous dose
- some 6–12 hours after transdermal application.

Analgesia lasts for 30–60 minutes after a single i.v. dose and up to 72 hours after a correctly applied transdermal patch.

THERAPEUTIC USES IN PAIN MANAGEMENT

- Fentanyl is widely used as a perioperative i.v. analgesic.
- The transdermal form of fentanyl has recently been introduced for the management of chronic cancer pain when opioid requirements are stable.

UNWANTED EFFECTS

Fentanyl is known to have a lower incidence of histamine release. Claims that it is less sedating and less constipating than morphine in chronic use have not yet been tested in clinical trials. Local erythema, itching and rash have been reported after the use of fentanyl patches.

> **Fentanyl is related to pethidine and should not be used in patients who have been on MAOIs in the previous 14 days.**

> **The use of transdermal fentanyl ('fentanyl patches') is absolutely contraindicated in acute pain: there have been fatalities when it has been given for postoperative pain.**

TRANSDERMAL FENTANYL

This has recently been introduced for cancer pain management in the UK. It is not suitable for use in patients with unstable opioid requirements as there is a long lag time (at least 2 hours) before an appreciable serum level of the drug is achieved, and the steady state is reached only after 12–24 hours. There is then a delay of some 16–24 hours, after the patch is removed, before the serum level of fentanyl falls significantly.

A fentanyl patch is a membrane-modulated system which allows more reliable transdermal delivery of the drug than an ointment or cream. After application a depot of drug will collect in the upper layer of the skin, so that it is then slowly available to the systemic circulation. A steady state is reached within 12–24 hours of application (typically about 14 hours), and remains at that level for 72 hours in the majority of patients (though there are reports of patients requiring another patch at 48 hours). Once equilibrium is reached the patch will maintain analgesic concentrations which are similar to those of an i.v. infusion.

During the time when the serum level of fentanyl is rising 'rescue' analgesia for breakthrough pain must be available: for most patients this will be oral morphine. If the patient can take oral normal-release morphine then he or she will be able to take a modified-release preparation, and therefore TTS-fentanyl will not be needed.

The present known indication for TTS-fentanyl is patients in chronic pain with stable opioid requirements who cannot or prefer not to take regular oral analgesia.

At present it is uncertain whether the advantages over morphine (better quality of sleep, less sedation, less constipation) reported in small groups of patients in open trials will be confirmed in larger, formal trials.

Possible indications are:

- patients on chronic, stable morphine therapy with severe constipation not helped by standard therapy
- patients on chronic, stable morphine therapy with disabling sedation.

Contraindications

Transdermal fentanyl must not be used in acute pain: the decline in serum drug levels after removal of the patch is considerably slower than after i.v. use (16–20 hours), probably because of continued absorption from a skin depot. If the pain has lessened in that period there is a grave danger of fatal respiratory depression.

Precautions

Overdosing has been reported when a heat pad has been placed over the fentanyl patch: any local heating will cause an increase in absorption of the drug, and the short duration of action (48 rather than 72 hours) of the patch in some patients has been attributed to cancer fever.

METHADONE

This is a powerful synthetic opioid which acts primarily through the μ receptor to produce analgesia, but which also has significant activity at the δ receptor. Recent work also suggests that methadone is an NMDA (*n*-methyl-D-aspartate) antagonist. There is no ceiling to its analgesic effects. One of its most important differences from morphine is its **prolonged half-life**, due to accumulation in chronic use. The use of methadone in pain management declined after several reports of apnoea in patients put on a fixed dosing schedule. It is now being favoured again in cancer pain management as an alternative to morphine, when that drug is ineffective or poorly tolerated.

Methadone is well absorbed from all routes of administration. Appreciable plasma concentrations are reached 30 minutes after oral administration. Oral bioavailability is about 80%.

Plasma half-life

The half-life of methadone varies considerably between individuals and, between single and multiple doses.

Methadone is a very lipophilic drug with a large volume of distribution. When a single dose is given the half-life is dependent on distribution into the tissues and renal and hepatic clearance. The half-life of a single oral dose varies from 12 to 18 hours (an i.m. dose from 6 to 8 hours). With continued use an extensive tissue reservoir of methadone is created, so that only 1% of the body stores of the drug are in the plasma. The half-life then becomes more dependent on clearance, as the tissue stores are partially filled. Methadone will be leached out of this accumulated tissue store and the half-life, in chronic use, may vary from 10 to 75 hours. A steady state will not be reached for 2–10 days after a change in dose in these circumstances. This makes it a difficult drug for the non-specialist to titrate. Methadone is also highly protein bound, which also contributes to its prolonged half-life.

The half life of methadone increases with age.

In acute pain analgesia will last for 4–6 hours. When methadone is used in chronic pain its accumulation will allow doses to be given less frequently. Analgesia generally lasts 6–12 hours, but the regimen must be adjusted to suit the individual and for the first 5–6 days at least the patient must be under very close medical supervision (see Chapter 14).

Metabolism

Metabolism takes place in the liver and there are no pharmacologically active metabolites.

THERAPEUTIC USES IN PAIN RELIEF

- As an alternative to morphine in the management of severe nociceptive pain, when morphine is causing intolerable side-effects
- As the analgesic of first choice in severe nociceptive pain in some centres (not in the UK)
- Its structure is so different from morphine that it can be used in patients who have a true allergy to that drug
- As an alternative to morphine, or other strong opioids, when these drugs are proving ineffective at very high dose
- In morphine-induced pain ('paradoxical pain').

When transferring a patient from morphine to methadone careful titration is needed, as a simple conversion to a calculated equianalgesic dose will often mean that too high a dose is given.

Contraindications

- Acute pain
- Obstetric patients
- The elderly
- The confused or demented patient
- Patients with hepatic or renal failure.

Precautions when using methadone

In high doses propranolol, phenothiazines and tricyclic antidepressants can all displace methadone from its plasma protein-binding sites, leading to a greater than expected pharmacological effect. Patients on these drugs should be closely monitored.

ADMINISTRATION

Oral

This is the best route for the administration of methadone. The oral solution is a viscous green liquid which cannot be used parenterally. It is very attractive to children and there have been several fatalities reported because childproof containers have not been used.

Rectal

Methadone is well absorbed rectally, and custom-made suppositories of up to 600 mg have been used. The limitations of this route apply, but it may be a good alternative where parenteral routes are not available.

Parenteral

- Methadone is irritant, so subcutaneous administration for long periods is not recommended.
- Methadone can be used intravenously or intramuscularly, with the usual precautions that apply when opioids are given in this way.
- It is not used intraspinally.

> **Because of its prolonged half-life repeated doses of naloxone, or a naloxone infusion, will be needed if an overdose of methadone has been taken.**

HYDROMORPHONE

Hydromorphone is a strong μ agonist suitable for the treatment of severe nociceptive pain (step 3 analgesic). It is 6–10 times more potent than morphine. It has been widely used in the USA for a number of years and is now available in the UK. Hydromorphone is well absorbed by the oral, rectal and parenteral routes, although it undergoes extensive first-pass metabolism. Its plasma half-life is only 2 hours, but analgesia may last 3–4 hours. When given intrathecally it causes less pruritus than morphine.

NALOXONE

Naloxone is a **pure opioid antagonist** which will occupy, and displace opioids from, all receptors, but with the greatest affinity for the μ receptor. It is used therapeutically to reverse respiratory depression caused by opioids, but will also reverse the analgesic and other effects of these drugs. Patients do not become tolerant to naloxone. Overdosage has not been reported. If given in standard doses to people who have not received opioids it has no known pharmacological effects.

Oral absorption

Naloxone cannot usefully be given by mouth as it is rapidly metabolized and inactivated. The oral to parenteral ratio has been estimated at 50:1.

Parenteral administration

Naloxone is given by the intravenous, subcutaneous or intramuscular routes.

Plasma half-life

This is 60–90 minutes in adults and up to 3 hours in neonates.

The onset of action is within:

- 1–2 minutes of i.v. administration
- 2–5 minutes of subcutaneous or i.m. administration.

The duration of its effect is anything between 15 and 90 minutes following i.v. administration: it may be longer after i.m. administration.

> **The duration of action of most opioids exceeds that of a standard single dose of naloxone, so frequent injections or an infusion of the drug may need to be given to treat an overdose effectively.**

Metabolism

Naloxone is rapidly metabolized in the liver, mostly by glucuronidation. The metabolites and some unchanged naloxone are excreted in the urine.

THERAPEUTIC USES IN PAIN MANAGEMENT

The primary use of naloxone is to reverse the unwanted respiratory depression caused either by an overdose of opioid or by an exaggerated individual response to an opioid. It has been reported that it will reverse the respiratory depression caused by spinal opioids without reversing analgesia. This is still a matter of controversy.

It has been used in the treatment of central (post-stroke) pain.

Unwanted effects

In standard doses, when the dose is titrated to produce a desired effect, naloxone has no unwanted effects.

> **The sudden reversal of analgesia in patients on opioids can produce dangerous cardiac dysrhythmias, pulmonary oedema and hypertension or hypotension.**

Many of these reported effects have occurred in postoperative patients with known pre-existing cardiac abnormalities given small doses of naloxone (100–400 μg). It is **essential** that naloxone is used with great caution in patients with **underlying pain** (or those physically dependent on opioids), as it is thought that the sudden reversal of analgesia produces an outpouring of catecholamines, which in turn leads to the adverse effects on the cardiovascular system. When naloxone is used to reverse respiratory depression in such patients the dose should be given extremely slowly and cautiously, so that the minimum amount of drug needed to produce the desired effect is used.

Precautions and contraindications

Naloxone is a very safe drug and there are no absolute contraindications to its use, but judgement must be used in the following circumstances:

- In all patients with pre-existing pain (see above), particularly those with known cardiac disease
- In all patients receiving cardiotoxic drugs
- It should not be the sole available method of resuscitating patients with respiratory depression following opioid overdose: other standard methods of resuscitation should be available, for example bag and mask ventilation.
- In patients who are physically dependent on opioids it will precipitate an acute withdrawal syndrome. Do not forget the babies of opioid-dependent mothers on these drugs throughout pregnancy.

Suggested starting doses

For postoperative respiratory depression start with 0.1–0.2 mg i.v. initially and repeat at 1–2-minute intervals according to the patient's response. If necessary an infusion can be set up, starting at 2.5 μg/kg/h, adjusted as necessary.

TRAMADOL

This drug has both opioid and non-opioid properties. It acts **centrally** at opioid receptors and is thought to affect the **descending inhibitory pathways** that modulate nociception, possibly by inhibiting presynaptic monoamine uptake and stimulating serotonin release.

It was introduced into UK practice in 1995 but has been used elsewhere in Europe for some years. Tramadol is effective in the management of moderately severe acute and chronic pain (a step 2 analgesic on the WHO ladder). It seems to have a low abuse potential and is not a controlled drug.

Tramadol can be given orally, intravenously, intramuscularly, subcutaneously and rectally. Analgesia lasts 3–4 hours after oral administration and 5–6 hours after being given i.m. There is little reported experience with high doses.

CHAPTER 4

NON-OPIOID ANALGESICS

This group includes aspirin, paracetamol and the other NSAIDs (non-steroidal anti-inflammatory drugs). These drugs exert their analgesic actions by both central and peripheral mechanisms.

Non-opioid analgesics

- have no activity at opioid receptor sites
- do not induce tolerance or dependence
- have a ceiling effect for analgesia.

All can be given orally and this is the most common route of administration. Others can be given rectally, topically, intramuscularly and subcutaneously.

These drugs are used in step 1 of the WHO Analgesic Pain Ladder (see Fig. 2.1), but when other drugs are started – morphine, for example – the non-opioid analgesic may often be continued with benefit.

PARACETAMOL (ACETAMINOPHEN, USA)

This synthetic non-opioid analgesic is the active metabolite of the more toxic phenacetin. Its mechanism of action, analgesic activity and antipyretic effect are similar to aspirin, but in contrast it has weak anti-inflammatory activity and a negligible effect on platelets.

Paracetamol also acts centrally, **inhibiting brain cyclo-oxygenase and nitric oxide synthase**.

Paracetamol has now overtaken aspirin in over-the-counter sales in the UK.

PHARMACOKINETICS

Paracetamol is usually administered orally, although it can be given by suppository. The rectal dose is some 30–40% higher than the oral dose because of reduced bioavailability.

Oral absorption

Paracetamol is rapidly and almost completely absorbed from the upper GI tract.

The plasma half-life is 2–3 hours and, peak analgesia occurs within 30–60 minutes.

Metabolism

This occurs in the liver and the metabolites, mostly sulphates and glucuronides, are excreted in the urine. The metabolic pathways are saturable, and this explains the incidence of hepatic necrosis in overdose.

THERAPEUTIC USES IN PAIN RELIEF

Paracetamol is used in the management of mild to moderate pain for both acute and chronic conditions. It does not have some of the adverse effects of aspirin (such as gastropathy), and may be used safely in patients for whom salicylates are contraindicated.

Contraindications

In normal use paracetamol is very safe. As with all drugs anaphylaxis can occur, though it is very rare, and paracetamol should not be given to people who have demonstrated sensitivity to it. Cross-sensitivity in people who are allergic to aspirin has been reported, but the incidence is probably less than 5%.

Acute toxicity

Dose-dependent acute toxicity leads to hepatic failure, which can be fatal (it is responsible for about 160 deaths per annum in the UK), and has led to calls for restrictions on the use of paracetamol. At therapeutic doses a minor route of paracetamol metabolism is its conversion by hepatic cytochrome P450-dependent microsomal oxidase. The metabolite formed by this path is highly reactive, but normally inactivated by conjugation with glutathione. If sufficient paracetamol is taken glutathione is depleted and the metabolite binds covalently to hepatic proteins, causing necrosis. Toxicity is very unlikely with recommended doses (4–6 g/day), although some people will be more susceptible to toxicity than others because:

- they have a greater reliance on the microsomal oxidation pathway for genetic reasons
- the metabolic pathway has been stimulated by simultaneous use of enzyme-inducing drugs such as anticonvulsants or alcohol
- they have chronic alcoholic liver disease.

Chronic toxicity

Nephropathy has been reported with long-term use of analgesics: it is thought to be associated with **combined preparations**, especially those that contain phenacetin. Although it has not been reported with paracetamol alone, the indications for the use of any drug in the longterm should be regularly reviewed because of possible toxicity.

Dosage

The *British National Formulary* recommends 1 g every 6 hours, although 1 g every 4 hours is commonly prescribed on palliative care units.

ASPIRIN

Aspirin can be regarded as the parent NSAID. Structurally it is a semisynthetic derivative of naturally occurring salicyclic acid, and is classed as a salicylate. In the body aspirin is hydrolysed to salicylate and acetate. The salicylate component appears to be responsible for its therapeutic properties, which are:

- analgesia at all doses
- antipyretic effect in feverish patients at all doses
- anti-inflammatory effect when used in doses above 3.6 g daily.

Its mechanisms of action are not fully understood, but it is well established that it **irreversibly** inhibits acetylating cyclo-oxygenase, which converts arachidonic acid into cyclic endoperoxides. Through its effects on prostaglandin synthesis aspirin has actions throughout the body (Table 4.1)

TABLE 4.1 The effects of aspirin on the body

System	*Effects*	*Notes*
Haematological	Prolongs bleeding time Inhibits platelet aggregation	Effect lasts for lifetime of the platelet (about 10 days). Reversed when new platelets made after aspirin stopped
Genitourinary/renal	Inhibition of uterine contractions Dose-dependent uricosuric effect Decreases renal blood flow (RBF)	Effect on RBF greatest in those with renal impairment or salt and water retention: avoid in these patients
CVS	Dilatation of peripheral blood vessels	Large doses only
Respiratory/metabolic	Respiratory stimulation by peripheral/central mechanisms Uncoupling of oxidative phosphorylation	Toxic doses
CNS	Inhibit the synthesis/release of prostaglandins that mediate effect of endogenous pyrogen in the hypothalamus	

Aspirin is being overtaken by paracetamol as the standard mild analgesic because of its potentially serious adverse effects.

Aspirin is very commonly bought over the counter and consumed either alone or in combination with other drugs. It may not be apparent from the drug name (e.g. Alka-Seltzer) that the preparation contains aspirin.

PHARMACOKINETICS

Aspirin is rapidly hydrolysed in the body to salicyclic acid and acetate. It can be given orally or rectally. After an oral dose it is rapidly and completely absorbed from the stomach and upper small intestine.

Plasma half-life is 15–20 minutes.

Peak analgesia occurs between 15 minutes and 2 hours after administration, the difference depending on the formulation and dose used.

Analgesia lasts 4–6 hours.

Metabolism

After oral administration aspirin is partially hydrolysed to salicylate by esterases in the GI mucosa while being absorbed. After absorption remaining unhydrolysed aspirin is converted to salicylate, principally in the liver but also in plasma, erythrocytes and synovial fluid.

THERAPEUTIC USES IN PAIN RELIEF

Aspirin is the parent drug of step 1 of the WHO Pain Ladder, being used in both acute and chronic pain. It is particularly useful in inflammatory conditions, although in current practice another NSAID would often be prescribed for this indication.

Unwanted effects

The gastrointestinal tract

The most serious effect is GI bleeding. All patients taking aspirin have detectable blood loss in the stool: it is usually symptomless and is the result of a local effect on the GI mucosa. Possible lesions include erythema, petechiae, submucosal bleeding erosions and ulceration. Bleeding and other symptoms may be present, but even quite severe damage may be silent for a time. Some patients using long-term aspirin at normal doses develop iron-deficiency anaemia.

Major GI bleeds may occur in patients on aspirin – they are not uncommon and cannot be predicted from the degree of occult blood loss that has gone before.

Other GI symptoms which may occur in patients on aspirin include:

- dyspepsia and heartburn
- nausea and, more rarely, vomiting. These occur through both a local effect on gastric mucosa and a central effect at higher doses.

These minor GI symptoms occur more commonly at higher doses and may be reduced by taking the aspirin with food or large quantities of milk or antacid.

Peptic ulcer formation

Aspirin causes gastric mucosal damage ranging from erythema to frank ulceration. Latent or old peptic ulceration can also be reactivated. Neither enteric-coated formulations nor buffered tablets appear to protect against these hazards.

The ear

Aspirin has effects on the inner ear, causing tinnitus in those on chronic therapy or taking large doses. Hearing loss can also result. Both of these effects are usually completely reversible when the drug is withdrawn, although some cases of permanent hearing loss have been reported.

Sensitivity reactions

These are more common in people with atopy (20% of patients with chronic urticaria) than in the general population (0.3%). They take the form of:

- bronchospasm: 4% of people with asthma show a sensitivity reaction to aspirin. These patients more commonly have nasal polyps. The bronchospasm typically develops 15–30 minutes after ingestion of the drug and may be extremely mild or very serious requiring hospital in-patient treatment. Patients sometimes develop this after taking aspirin for some years with no problems
- anaphylactic/anaphylactoid reactions: these may require treatment with adrenaline, steroids and antihistamines, as well as general supportive measures
- urticaria and angio-oedema: these occurs most frequently in patients with chronic urticaria and chronic rhinitis.

> **Aspirin is contraindicated in any patient who demonstrates sensitivity to another NSAID, and vice versa, as cross-sensitivity is common.**

PRECAUTIONS AND CONTRAINDICATIONS

Aspirin should be used cautiously if at all in the following groups of patients:

- Those with established peptic ulceration or a history of GI bleeding
- Those with renal impairment, as aspirin is largely excreted in the urine and these patients are also at risk of unwanted renal effects
- Those with a bleeding diathesis related to either disease or drug therapy
- Those about to undergo surgery: aspirin should be discontinued at least 1 week before a surgical procedure to allow the manufacture of new platelets.

Paediatric precautions

The CSM (Committee on Safety of Medicines) has recommended that aspirin not be given to children under the age of 12 years because of the risk of their developing Reye's syndrome. Under expert guidance it is still prescribed for serious diseases such as juvenile chronic arthritis.

Pregnancy and lactation

Low-dose aspirin seems to be safe in pregnancy. The safety of analgesic or anti-inflammatory doses of aspirin is doubtful.

Drug interactions

There are many drug interactions involving aspirin, and it is safest to check a formulary before prescribing it. The most important clinically are:

- interaction with anticoagulants: because of its effects on platelets and its potential to cause GI bleeding aspirin should not be used in conjunction with anticoagulants
- interactions with uricosuric agents: salicylates will inhibit the effect of uricosuric drugs, and they should not be taken together regularly
- interaction with hypoglycaemic agents: the hypoglycaemic effect of the sulphonylureas is enhanced
- interaction with methotrexate (MTX): the toxicity of methotrexate is potentiated when used with aspirin because renal excretion of MTX is reduced and because it is displaced from its plasma protein-binding sites.

ADMINISTRATION

Oral aspirin

Aspirin is usually administered orally, and it is preferable to take it with food, water or milk to reduce the possibility of gastric irritation.

Oral preparations

There is a widely held theory that the smaller the particle size in the preparation the more rapidly the aspirin is absorbed and the less the gastrotoxicity. However, there is no evidence to support this. There is no research which has clearly demonstrated that the formulation of aspirin is important in reducing GI bleeding at normal therapeutic doses: minimizing the dose is likely to be most important.

Definitions

Soluble aspirin BP The calcium carbonate and citric acid which are combined with aspirin in this combination react with water and effervesce, so the aspirin is dispersed into a fine suspension. This is said to allow more rapid absorption, so that high local concentrations are minimized.

Buffered tablets These are mixtures of aspirin and antacids. In theory there is less mucosal damage associated with buffered aspirin, as gastric acidity is reduced by the antacid component. This has not been confirmed by research.

Enteric-coated aspirin The aspirin is released in the small intestine where the environment is relatively alkaline, which should prevent local damage to gastric mucosa although duodenal damage will be possible. Again research findings have not verified this.

Modified-release aspirin A diffusion-polymer coating means that the aspirin is released slowly in the intestine over a 4-hour period. This has no clinical relevance, as there may only be a significant reduction in blood loss at doses above 4 g of aspirin daily, which should not be used. The usual dose of aspirin is 300–900 mg every 4–6 hours. No more than 4 g should be given in one day.

Rectal administration

Absorption may be slow or incomplete, and a larger dose is needed. The extent of absorption increases with the length of time that the suppository is retained.

Give 2–3 suppositories every 4 hours to a maximum of 12 in a 24-hour period.

BENORYLATE

This ester of paracetamol and aspirin is hydrolysed after absorption to its two constituent drugs. It need only be given twice daily.

THE NSAIDs

This is a large, heterogeneous group of compounds with the defining characteristics that they are all **weakly acidic, highly protein bound** and **naloxone insensitive**. They are extremely commonly used: there are 20 million prescriptions per year for NSAIDs in the UK and 1.2% of the population of the USA are taking one regularly. Many are available over the counter.

NSAIDs can be grouped by similarities in chemical structure but this cannot be used as a guide to their analgesic efficacy. If a patient tries one and does not receive good pain relief or suffers unacceptable unwanted effects, then it is not uncommon for another to be tried and perhaps a third or fourth before a suitable one is selected. There is no rationale for making the selection on the basis of a different chemical structure.

ANALGESIC ACTION

The role of cyclo-oxygenase

Prostaglandins **sensitize** and **activate peripheral nociceptors** to mechanical stress and pain mediators such as histamine and bradykinin. The formation of prostaglandins is catalysed by the enzyme cyclo-oxygenase (COX), which is now known to exist in two forms, COX -1 and COX-2. COX-1 is found normally in many tissues (the stomach, kidneys and platelets, for example), whereas COX-2 is found mainly after induction by vasoactive hormones, endotoxins, certain cytokines, mitogens and growth factors. Analgesic activity is not related to the potency of any NSAID as an in vitro cyclo-oxygenase inhibitor, although anti-inflammatory actions are. There is a differential inhibition of COX-1 and COX-2 by different NSAIDs, and this may help to explain the varying adverse effects of the drugs. **Present evidence suggests that the anti-inflammatory and antinociceptive activities of NSAIDs are dissociated**. It is hoped that the development of selective COX-2 inhibitors, to replace NSAIDs, will allow the analgesic actions to be separated from the unwanted effects secondary to the inhibition of COX-1. There is as yet insufficient evidence to support this hypothesis.

The analgesic effects of the NSAIDs are likely to be related to:

- COX inhibition: prostaglandins may sensitize nociceptors to pain mediators such as histamine and bradykinin. NSAIDs may reduce pain in inflammatory conditions by inhibiting COX, and hence the formation of prostaglandins
- Interaction with endogenous opioid systems: it has been shown that NSAIDs reach the CSF after oral administration. Although they do not have effects at opioid receptors, NSAIDs may interact with endogenous opioid systems to enhance analgesia

- inhibition of neutrophil activation: it has been proposed that this may play a part in the anti-inflammatory and analgesic activity of NSAIDs
- activity at spinal level: this activity is probably independent of their actions on prostaglandins, and may be related to the NMDA receptor and the inhibition of 'wind-up'. It may be related to inhibition of nitric oxide synthase in the spinal cord.

PHARMACOKINETICS

All NSAIDs are well absorbed from the upper GI tract by passive diffusion, and appreciable plasma levels are reached 30 minutes after administration, with levels peaking at about 2 hours for most drugs. Different preparations will have different absorption characteristics: for example, many drugs exist in enteric-coated or modified-release forms.

All NSAIDs are highly protein bound to serum albumin – typically this is greater than 90%. It is the non-bound fraction which is pharmacologically active, and many patients with chronic illness taking NSAIDs have low serum albumin and a greater portion of the NSAID in the unbound active form.

Most NSAIDs undergo enterohepatic circulation, which helps explain why **the route of administration is not relevant in the production of gastropathy**.

NSAIDs are not disease-altering drugs, and so the potential of an NSAID to cause morbidity and mortality in an individual weighs in the selection of the drug.

THERAPEUTIC USES IN PAIN RELIEF

- In the inflammatory arthropathies, such as rheumatoid arthritis, and the connective tissue diseases such as SLE
- Cancer pain, particularly bony metastases
- Renal and biliary colic
- Osteoarthritis, although in many patients, especially the elderly, the best first-line treatment would be regular paracetamol, which has a much lower incidence of unwanted effects
- Gout
- Bursitis
- Soft tissue injuries
- Postoperative analgesia, both parenterally and orally
- Primary dysmenorrhea; this is probably related to inhibition of prostaglandins or modulation of their effects
- Low back pain
- Headache and migraine.

Haematological effects

Platelet aggregation is inhibited and the bleeding time prolonged while a patient is taking NSAIDs. This effect is reversible, lasting only as long as an effective blood concentration of the drug exists, and is thought to be related to COX-1 inhibition.

It must be remembered that the bleeding time will be *prolonged until the NSAID has been excreted*. This will take five half-lives of the drug. Adequate time must be left before surgery.

Gastrointestinal effects

NSAIDs have the following known effects on the stomach and duodenum:

- Dyspepsia, which is the most frequently occurring adverse effect that is reported to the CSM
- Symptomless gastric erosions: endoscopy has revealed that this may occur in 20–40% of patients on NSAIDs
- Gastroduodenal ulceration: this may have an incidence of 10–30% in patients on NSAIDs
- Gastroduodenal perforation
- Gastroduodenal haemorrhage: the risk is estimated to be three times greater for someone on NSAIDs than for an untreated control, and the mortality increases with age.

Perforation and haemorrhage can occur in any part of the GI tract.

Chronic use is also associated with:

- small and large bowel strictures, especially when modified-release forms are used for a year or more. Intestinal obstruction may complicate these strictures, which are irreversible
- Exacerbation of existing colitis
- Precipitation of de novo colitis
- 'NSAID enteropathy' protein loss, leading to hypoalbuminaemia, low-grade inflammation and microscopic bleeding.

There are various theories to explain the aetiology of this damage to the GI tract:

- Reduction in protective barrier: the stomach produces prostaglandins, which are involved in the production of mucus and bicarbonate and regulating microvascular blood flow. If this protective barrier is reduced the mucosa becomes susceptible to damage by H^+ions
- Increase in intestinal permeability: NSAIDs appear to damage enterocyte mitochondria during absorption by uncoupling oxidative phosphorylation. A cascade of effects then follows which leads to both an increase in intestinal permeability and the production of damaging oxidative species.

Similar mechanisms also increase the susceptibilty of the colon to secondary damage induced by luminal toxins and bacteria.

Prevention of NSAID- induced injury to the bowel

- Prescribe one of the NSAIDs that current evidence suggests is least likely to cause toxicity: it is clear that some drugs are more toxic to the gut than others (see below).
- Prescribe the drug at the **lowest possible dose for the shortest possible time**.
- Keep necessary chronic use under review.
- Ask whether a less toxic class of drug (for example paracetamol in osteoarthritis) could be used in high-risk individuals.
- Ask about bowel symptoms when reviewing the patient, and consider changing/stopping the drug if these occur, but remember peptic ulceration is often silent.
- Prescribe misoprostol and/or H_2 receptor antagonists or proton pump inhibitors concurrently with NSAIDs in high-risk individuals.

A drug with low gut toxicity is ibuprofen.
Drugs with intermediate toxicity are diclofenac and naproxen.
Drugs with very high toxicity are piroxicam and azapropazone.

Renal effects of NSAIDs

The NSAIDs are associated with a number of adverse effects on the kidneys, although most are rare. The kidney produces PGI_2, PGE_2 and some $PGF_{2\alpha}$. These are involved in local modulation of renal blood flow, glomerular filtration rate, renin release, the concentrating mechanism for urine and the excretion of sodium and potassium. The unwanted effects of NSAIDs result from the decrease in production of these prostaglandins, and are summarized below.

1. Acute reversible/vasomotor renal failure
2. Interference with the renal excretion of:
   - water
   - sodium
   - potassium.
3. Interference with:
   - antihypertensive therapy
   - diuretic therapy.
4. Acute interstitial nephritis with or without renal failure
5. Nephrotic syndrome with or without interstitial nephritis, with or without renal failure
6. Chronic renal injury, 'analgesic nephropathy'.

CNS effects

It is known that NSAIDs cross into the CNS and a wide range of unwanted effects have been reported, including:

- headaches
- exacerbation of Parkinson's disease (with sulindac, naproxen and flurbiprofen, for example)
- extrapyramidal symptoms, including oculogyric crises, tremor and dystonic reactions
- confusion (especially with indomethacin)
- cognitive impairment
- giddiness (most commonly with indomethacin).

Respiratory effects

NSAIDs can precipiate an attack of asthma in people who suffer from this disease. It is more likely in those with aspirin-sensitive asthma.

Pregnancy and lactation

There are specific risks associated with NSAIDs in pregnancy. In the third trimester their use has been associated with premature closure of the ductus arteriosus in the neonate. Uterine contraction may be inhibited during labour. Their excretion into breast milk has caused cyanotic crises in the newborn.

PRECAUTIONS AND CONTRAINDICATIONS (Table 4.2)

The following conditions increase the risk of a patient suffering an unwanted effect from an NSAID:

- Advancing age: this is an independent risk factor for the development of gastrointestinal complications of NSAIDs and fatal haemorrhage is more likely to occur in this age group. Over the age of 75 years the risk is increased fivefold. Renal complications are also more common.

- A previous history of peptic ulceration.
- Corticosteroid use: gives a fourfold risk of peptic ulceration.
- Use of anticoagulants: the patient is at greater risk of dangerous bleeding if an NSAID is started.
- Long-term therapy is associated with a higher risk of all the GI and renal complications of NSAIDs.
- The use of diuretics, and other salt-depleted states, leads to a greater risk of the renal complications of NSAIDs.
- Hepatic cirrhosis with or without ascites increases the risk of both renal and hepatic complications of NSAIDs.
- Extensive atherosclerosis: renal complications of NSAIDs are more likely, and a bleeding complication will be more risky for those with cardiac disease.
- Renal impairment.
- Congestive cardiac failure: greater risk of acute tubular necrosis.
- Myeloma: these patients have an increased risk of renal failure.

Table 4.2 NSAID interactions

Drug affected	*Effect*
Anticoagulants, warfarin	Inhibition of metabolism
Antidiabetics, sulphonylureas	Enhanced effect
Antiepileptics, phenytoin	Enhanced effect due to increased plasma displacement
Antihypertensives	Antagonism of effect, risk of hyperkalaemia, increased risk of renal failure on administration of captopril
Cardiac glycosides, filtration	Exacerbation of heart failure, reduced glomerular rate and increased digoxin concentration
Diuretics, effect	Increased risk of nephrotoxicity and reduction in diuretic
Methotrexate	Excretion delayed

From Kaufman and Jahemer 1996 Pharmacology in the practice of anaesthesia. Edward Arnold, with permission

DRUG ADMINISTRATION

Oral

This is the most common route of administration and is to be preferred in acute and chronic use. In any condition where NSAID toxicity is more likely, such as renal impairment, close monitoring of the patient is necessary and dosage reductions should be made where appropriate.

Rectal

It is important to remember that the following have been reported with all NSAID suppositories:

- rectal irritation
- proctitis
- rectal ulceration
- formation of strictures.

The rectal dose is likely to be 30–40% higher because of reduced bioavailability by this route.

Parenteral

Diclofenac, ketoprofen and ketorolac can all be given by injection. The first two are given by deep intramuscular injection, which minimizes tissue damage. Ketorolac can be given subcutaneously and intravenously, but the CSM recommends that parenteral use does not exceed 2 days and it is absolutely contraindicated in anyone with a bleeding disorder.

Intramuscular injections of NSAIDs are used in:

- postoperative pain control
- treatment of renal colic.

> **Remember:** If a patient can take oral medication there is no advantage in giving an NSAID intramuscularly as the time to analgesia is the same by any route: i.m. diclofenac is both painful and associated with the formation of abscesses.

Transdermal

e.g. benzydamine, diclofenac, felbinac, ibuprofen, ketoprofen and piroxicam.

There is now evidence to suggest that this route of administration is associated with **fewer unwanted gastrointestinal effects**. One explanation of this is the concept of 'local enhanced topical delivery' (LETD). The drug reaches a target tissue by direct diffusion and accumulates there in greater concentration than could have been achieved by oral or parenteral administration. Concentrations are higher in the skin and adjacent structures (e.g. muscle) than in deeper ones, e.g. synovial membrane or plasma. Therefore transdermal NSAIDs are most likely to be useful in soft-tissue injuries, when the gel is applied to the painful site, rather than in arthritic conditions.

NSAIDs should not be applied to damaged or unhealthy skin and should not be given to people with known hypersensitivity or a previous adverse reaction. Skin reactions are rare.

CHAPTER 5

LOCAL ANAESTHETICS

Local anaesthetics are a group of compounds which can produce **reversible local analgesia**: they do not affect the patient's level of consciousness. Their reversibility is a key part of their usefulness: many drugs have local anaesthetic properties but cause nerve damage. It is still not clearly established how local anaesthetics work, but it is known that they inhibit sodium flux in, and hence depolarization of, nerve endings, so that nerve transmission is inhibited in **sensory, motor and autonomic fibres**. Indeed, local anaesthetics affect **all excitable membranes**, which explains their cardiac and CNS toxicity. A knowledge of their adverse effects is important as their consequences may be fatal.

USES OF LOCAL ANAESTHETICS

Structurally, local anaesthetics follow a basic pattern of a lipophilic aromatic portion, an intermediate chain and a hydrophilic amine group. The intermediate group may have an amide or an ester linkage, which both gives the name to the two main classes of these drugs and explains important differences in their clinical pharmacology.

The important clinically significant pharmacological actions of local anaesthetics can be summarized as follows:

- A **reversible** block of nerve conduction in all types of nerve fibre and nerve ending
- Smooth muscle relaxation which leads to vasodilatation, for example
- A quinidine-like effect on cardiac conduction
- Mixed features of both stimulation (for example convulsions) and depression (for example coma) of the CNS; the predominant effect is dependent on dose and the agent being used.

Local anaesthetics will affect all nerve fibres, but the smallest-diameter nerves are the most sensitive to their effects. This means that autonomic nerve fibres will be blocked first, then somatic sensory nerves carrying pain, and then somatic motor fibres (Figure 5.1).

The concentration of a local anaesthetic solution and the drug used will also affect the types of nerve fibre blocked (Table 5.1). For example, bupivacaine 0.75% will cause complete motor blockade.

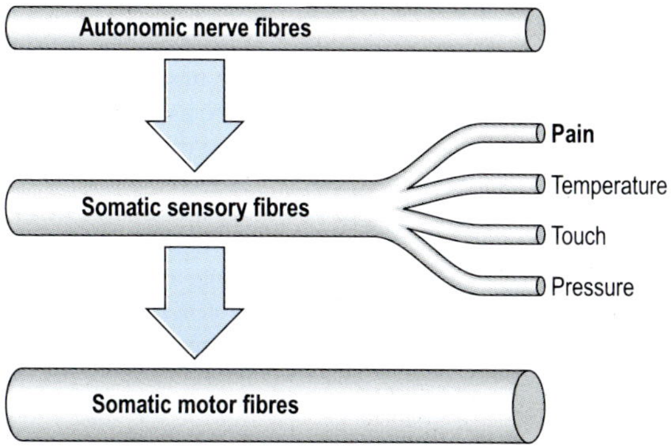

Fig. 5.1 Sensitivity of nerve fibres to blockade by local anaesthetic, the most susceptible fibres first.

TABLE 5.1 Differences between the esters and the amides

Amides	*Esters*
e.g. bupivacaine, lignocaine, prilocaine	e.g. amethocaine, cocaine, procaine hydrochloride
Most common injected anaesthetics	Most common topical anaesthetics
Metabolized by liver amidases	Metabolized by tissue esterases
Effect terminated by uptake into general circulation, therefore duration partly dependent on local blood flow	Effect terminated by metabolism, prolonged in hepatic failure as esterases synthesized in liver
Low incidence of allergy	High incidence of allergy

CHARACTERISTICS OF LOCAL ANAESTHETIC AGENTS

POTENCY

In the laboratory the potency of a local anaesthetic agent is directly proportional to its degree of lipid solubility, as to be effective the drug must penetrate the nerve membrane, which is 80% lipid. In clinical practice both potency and duration of action are also affected by the vasodilatory properties of the drug, as these will affect local blood flow.

Duration of action

The duration of action of local anaesthetic is also affected by its degree of protein binding, as this governs the rate at which the drug is released from its receptor sites in the nerve membrane. A drug such as bupivacaine, which is highly protein bound, is released slowly and has a more prolonged analgesic effect than prilocaine.

The unwanted effects of a highly protein-bound drug are more prolonged as well. Bupivacaine (96% protein bound) is contraindicated for intravenous regional anaesthesia (a Bier's block for example), as there have been fatalities from cardiac toxicity following tourniquet failure and escape of bupivacaine into the general circulation.

Addition of vasoconstrictors

Vasoconstrictor drugs are sometimes added to local anaesthetic agents to prolong their duration of action. They effect this by counteracting the vasodilatory effects of local anaesthetics, so that:

- the drug remains in contact with the nerve sheath for longer and more local anaesthetic is absorbed into it
- the rate of absorption of the local anaesthetic into the general circulation, and thus its metabolism, is slowed.

Vasoconstrictors have the greatest effect on short-lived drugs with pronounced vasodilatory properties: for example, the duration of action of lignocaine is substantially increased (see below) but prilocaine is little affected. Felypressin and adrenaline are the most commonly used vasoconstrictors in the UK.

Adrenaline

Adrenaline is usually added in a concentration of 5 μg/ml (1:200 000).

Felypressin

This is an analogue of the pituitary hormone oxytocin. It has no adrenergic effects and produces local vasoconstriction by a hormonal mechanism.

TOXICITY OF LOCAL ANAESTHETICS

Most unwanted effects of local anaesthetics results from an excessive plasma concentration of the drug, which results in CNS and/or cardiac toxicity. A high plasma concentration can occur when:

- too high a dose is administered to a given individual. **Quoted safe dose ranges are only a guide, and toxicity can result even when these are adhered to**.
- a bolus of drug is given directly into the general circulation, for example by unintentional intravascular injection, tourniquet failure in a Bier's block, or infiltration into a vascular area
- there is impaired metabolism of the drug; this can happen in patients with poor hepatic function or low hepatic blood flow.

Other unwanted effects associated with local anaesthetics include:

- drug allergy/hypersensitivity reaction
- the introduction of local anaesthetic into the wrong body compartment: for example, if a dose appropriate for epidural use is introduced into the subarachnoid space, caudal migration of the drug will result in anaesthesia of the medullary cardiac and respiratory centres, which will cause cardiac and respiratory collapse
- the effects of additives in the local anaesthetic solution.

CNS effects

These are dose dependent. At the lower end of the toxic dose range patients will experience symptoms of CNS stimulation: they may complain of feeling apprehensive, anxious, restless, nervous, confused and disorientated. Some patients will have convulsions.

At yet higher doses patients will experience CNS depression: drowsiness and eventually respiratory arrest will occur.

The pattern of toxicity is not fixed, and with lignocaine, for example, CNS stimulation may be fleeting and CNS depression more important.

CVS effects

Local anaesthetics share some properties with class 1 antidysrhythmic agents (quinidine is the prototype) and therefore in large doses, can depress the contractility of cardiac muscle causing hypotension and cardiac failure as well as precipitating dysrhythmias leading, if untreated, to cardiac arrest. Bupivacaine is especially important in this context (see below), and drug toxicity can be compounded by the other pharmacological effects of local anaesthetics on the cardiovascular and respiratory systems.

TREATMENT OF TOXICITY

Any clinician administering a local anaesthetic drug must be able to institute appropriate resuscitation in the event of an unwanted drug reaction. This may include the specific treatment of seizures and dysrhythmias, as well as general supportive measures.

- Vasodilatation and hypotension: the sympathetic vasomotor nerves are blocked when intraspinal local anaesthetic is used which can cause profound hypotension – the risk is greatest with intrathecal blockade. This unwanted effect will require preventative measures (i.v. fluids), active monitoring and sometimes specific treatment.
- Respiratory depression: can also follow from an **overdose** of intraspinal local anaesthetic. Cephalad spread of the drug can lead to block of the cardiac and respiratory centres in the brainstem: supportive therapy (i.v. fluids, intubation and artificial ventilation) must be instituted immediately and maintained until the effects of the local anaesthetic have worn off.

Effects of additives

Vasoconstrictors

When administered into the intravascular compartment these can cause dysrhythmias and hypertension: this can happen with unintentional intravenous injection during epidurals, for example.

> **Solutions containing vasoconstrictors should never be used in areas that receive a single blood supply (for example digits, ears, toes, the nose, the penis), as they may cause ischaemic damage, even gangrene. Such formulations should never be given systemically.**

Other additives

Local anaesthetic preparations may contain bacteriostatic agents (for example methylparaben) and preservatives (for example bisulphite), and these have been associated with neurotoxicity.

Local effects

When local anaesthetics are infiltrated into the skin they often cause a transient stinging or burning sensation. High concentrations of lignocaine used intrathecally may be neurotoxic.

PRECAUTIONS AND CONTRAINDICATIONS

- Anyone using a local anaesthetic must be familiar with its clinical pharmacology and potential problems associated with its use.
- When injecting local anaesthetic drugs the clinician should aspirate frequently to ensure that a blood vessel is not entered.
- The dose of local anaesthetic should be calculated with known safe dose ranges in mind and for the individual: for example, reduced doses should be given to the very elderly or those with hepatic impairment, as the rate of drug metabolism will be reduced.
- Vasoconstrictors are potentially more hazardous in patients with severe cardiac disease or other conditions associated with cardiovascular disease (for example diabetes), and the risks and benefits of using them should be carefully weighed.

Pregnancy

All local anaesthetics will cross the placenta but the amount that reaches the fetus will depend on the route by which the drug is given, the drug used and the dose administered. An experienced clinician must make these decisions in conjunction with the patient. Bupivacaine is preferred for parturients as it crosses the placenta in the smallest amount. Neurobehavioural changes (albeit subtle and short-lived) have been described in infants whose mothers were given mepivacaine or lignocaine in labour.

COMMONLY USED LOCAL ANAESTHETICS

ESTERS

Cocaine

This is the only local anaesthetic in current use which **vasoconstricts** because it blocks the reuptake of noradrenaline into nerve endings. This also results in potentiation of the effects of circulating catecholamines. If cocaine reaches the systemic circulation it causes CNS and CVS stimulation (it is a well known drug of addiction). It is only used topically now, mostly in ENT surgery.
Maximum recommended dose is 3 mg/kg

Amethocaine

This is commonly used in the USA as a spinal anaesthetic, but it has recently been developed as a gel which is becoming the most useful topical anaesthetic for intact skin. Unlike EMLA cream, its main rival, 4% amethocaine gel is relatively lipid soluble so that it is well absorbed into its site of action, the stratum corneum. In addition it causes local erythema and vasodilatation, thereby facilitating venepucture, and it has a more rapid onset of action than EMLA.

AMIDES

Lignocaine

This is the oldest amide anaesthetic in use. It is often used with the addition of adrenaline, as it has pronounced vasodilator activity and a relatively short duration.

Routes of administration

Subcutaneous infiltration, peripheral nerve blocks, intraspinal anaesthesia, as a gel for anaesthesia of mucous membranes (e.g. gel instilled into the urethra for urinary catheterization, for example).

Onset of analgesia

This is relatively rapid – within 3–5 minutes of infiltration.

Duration of analgesia

Plain lignocaine has an intermediate duration of action, but the addition of adrenaline makes it long-acting for local infiltration etc. It will not affect duration when lignocaine is used intravenously for other therapeutic purposes, and this would be extremely hazardous.

Maximum recommended doses are 3 mg/kg of plain solution and **7 mg/kg of a solution with additional adrenaline**.

Prilocaine

The anaesthetic effect of this drug is equipotent with lignocaine, but it is both less toxic and a less powerful vasodilator. In high doses (>10 mg/kg) one of its metabolites can cause methaemoglobinaemia: this is usually not significant though it is commoner in neonates; if necessary it can be treated with 1–2 mg/kg of methylene blue.

Routes of administration

Prilocaine may be used for nerve blocks, subcutaneous infiltration and intraspinal anaesthesia. It is the drug of choice for intravenous regional anaesthesia (e.g. Bier's blocks) because of its low toxicity.

Onset of analgesia occurs within 2 minutes of infiltration, and duration is approximately 1–2 hours.

Maximum recommended dose: plain solution 6 mg/kg; with adrenaline 8 mg/kg.

Bupivacaine

This is the longest-acting local anaesthetic drug currently available. It is favoured for regional anaesthesia (such as epidurals) following surgery, where a prolonged analgesic effect helps postoperative recovery. Its toxic effects are similarly prolonged because it is so highly tissue bound. Cardiac toxicity is the main hazard associated with its use and, as well as the cardiovascular depression seen with all local anaesthetics, ventricular tachycardia and fibrillation can occur.

Routes of administration
Infiltration, nerve blocks, intraspinal techniques.

> **The use of bupivacaine in intravenous regional anaesthesia is absolutely contraindicated.**

Onset of analgesia is relatively slow, taking up to 10 minutes. Duration is prolonged, and 4–6 hours is not unusual.

Maximum recommended doses are: Plain solution 2 mg/kg; with adrenaline 3 mg/kg; by infusion or epidural, 2 mg/kg should not be exceeded in any 4-hour period.

Ropivacaine

This recently introduced drug is as long acting as bupivacaine but appears to have less cardiac and CNS toxicity. At doses equipotent to bupivacaine it produces less motor blockade.

Routes of administration
Infiltration, intraspinal, nerve blocks.

No maximum recommended dose is given by the manufacturers but guidance is given in the *BNF* for different procedures.

PLASMA CONCENTRATIONS RESULTING FROM DIFFERENT ROUTES OF ADMINISTRATION

The plasma concentration of anaesthetic agents achieved for a given dose by different routes are shown in Figure 5.2 with the lowest concentrations first.

EMLA cream

The skin is a very effective barrier to drug penetration (see Chapter 2), and to be absorbed and exert an effect a topical emulsion has to contain at least 20% of the local anaesthetic in the uncharged base form. A eutectic mixture is one which has a lower melting point than either of its constituents alone. EMLA cream is a *e*utectic *m*ixture of *l*ocal *a*naesthetics, and contains prilocaine and lignocaine which, when mixed together, form a liquid at room temperature. This means that the concentration of local anaesthetic in the emulsion

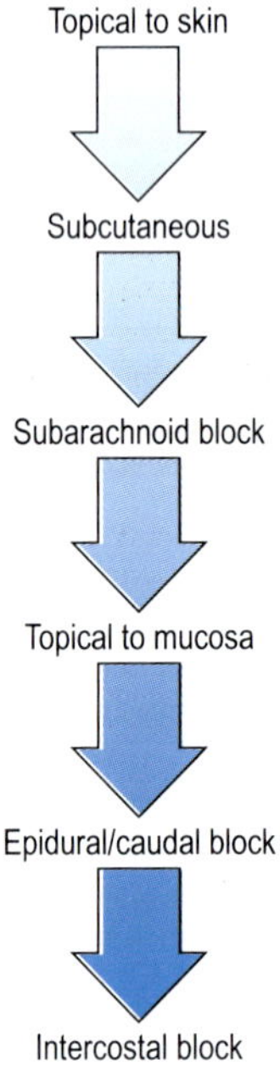

Fig. 5.2 Plasma concentrations of anaesthetic agents for a given dose by different routes.

droplets can be increased from 20% lignocaine in the plain emulsion to 80% in the lignocaine/prilocaine eutectic mixture, whereas the total concentration of local anaesthetic remains low. EMLA cream also contains an emulsifier, a viscosity-increasing agent and water (skin penetration is facilitated by aqueous solvents). 5% EMLA cream contains lignocaine 25 mg/g and prilocaine 25 mg/g.

Pharmacokinetics

EMLA cream must be applied **at least 1 hour** before its effects are needed, and preferably 1.5 hours. Its efficacy is in inverse proportion to dermal thickness.

Maximum plasma levels The maximum plasma level of anaesthetic is higher for lignocaine than for prilocaine, and is attained some 2–4 hours after application of the cream, depending where it is applied (for example, absorption from the face is more rapid than from the thicker skin on the forearm).

Toxic plasma concentrations of either drug have never been reported.

Duration of analgesia Analgesia increases during the first 2 hours after application of the cream and persists for 1–2 hours after its removal.

Therapeutic uses in pain relief

EMLA cream is principally used in the reduction of pain associated with venepuncture, mostly in children. Its use has been shown to increase compliance with the repeated venepuncture necessary for the effective treatment of some chronic childhood diseases.

EMLA has also been used for the relief of pain in a variety of medical and surgical procedures, such as:

- Lumbar puncture in children
- Arterial cannulation in adults and children; reduction of pain for cannulation in patients receiving haemodialysis
- Plastic surgery procedures, such as cutting split-skin grafts and punch skin biopsies
- Many other types of minor surgery and dermatological procedures
- The relief of refractory postherpetic neuralgia
- Prior to painful pain management procedures.

Unwanted effects

These are not usually clinically significant but mild, short-lived (1–2 hours) skin reactions have been reported, such as blanching and erythema, altered temperature sensation (so that washing with warm water is unpleasant) and itching. Its characteristic of causing skin blanching may make subsequent venepuncture more difficult.

Contraindications

EMLA is contraindicated in infants of less than 1 year because of the possibility of methaemoglobinaemia.

It should not be used in people who have a demonstrated allergy/hypersensitivity to either lignocaine or prilocaine.

Administration

It is important to allow sufficient time (an hour at least) for EMLA to take effect, and a thick layer should be applied, under an occlusive dressing, to the area to be anaesthetized.

CHAPTER 6

ANTIDEPRESSANTS AND ANTICONVULSANTS

THE ANTIDEPRESSANT DRUGS

Antidepressants are classified by the WHO as:

- tricyclics (TCADs)
- mianserin
- monoamine oxidase inhibitors (MAOIs)
- selective serotonin reuptake inhibitors (SSRIs)
- reversible inhibitors of monoamine oxidase A (RIMA).

All have some action on the nerve pathways mediated by **noradrenaline** (and other monoamines) and **serotonin** to **increase the concentrations of these neurotransmitters**. Descending inhibitory pathways from the brainstem (mediated by serotonin) and the midbrain (mediated by noradrenaline) are well described, and it has been shown that the antidepressants with mixed effects on both of these neurotransmitters are the most useful in pain relief. Antidepressants have at least three effects which help to contain pain in both chronic nonmalignant and cancer pain states:

- a direct analgesic effect of their own, particularly useful in neuropathic pain and tension headaches
- an 'opioid-sparing effect'
- their actions as antidepressant drugs.

PHARMACOLOGY OF TRICYCLIC ANTIDEPRESSANT DRUGS (TCADS)

Examples: amitriptyline, imipramine, lofepramine.

This group has very complex pharmacological actions which are not yet entirely understood. The term tricyclic antidepressant now encompasses drugs with 1, 2 and 4-ring structures which have a similar pharmacological spectrum. The general effect of these drugs is to **increase the concentration of various neurotransmitters in the CNS**, mostly by blocking the reuptake of serotonin and noradrenaline at the neuronal membrane. They also have powerful anticholinergic activity. Amitriptyline is still the most widely used in pain relief, although it has the important disadvantage of a high incidence of unwanted effects.

Remember:
- The adverse effects of these drugs appear within a few hours of administration.
- The analgesic effect appears within a few days.
- The antidepressant effect takes a few weeks (4–6 in most cases).

PHARMACOKINETICS

Absorption

Tricyclics are well absorbed by all routes of administration. Peak plasma concentrations vary enormously between individuals as a result of genetic differences in the speed of metabolism and degree of plasma protein binding. The relationship between plasma level and therapeutic effect is unclear and certainly not straightforward.

Oral absorption

Certain drugs (for example imipramine) undergo extensive first-pass metabolism when given by mouth.

THERAPEUTIC USES IN PAIN RELIEF

Neuropathic pain

Antidepressants, often in combination with anticonvulsants, are the drugs of choice for neuropathic pain (e.g. postherpetic neuralgia, neural injury by a malignant tumour). At many centres a TCAD is the drug of first choice, especially when the pain has a burning quality. A recent systematic review has shown no differences between anticonvulsants and antidepressants in the management of neuropathic pain.

Depression

Depression is an almost universal event during the course of many types of chronic illness, including cancer and chronic non-malignant pain. It is not always appropriate or necessary to treat it pharmacologically, but because of their dual action antidepressants may be particularly useful when both are present. The antidepressant action takes longer to come into effect and is only achieved at much higher doses. For example, in a well-nourished 30-year-old 150 mg nocte of amitriptyline might be required to achieve an antidepressant effect, but 50 mg nocte may have an appreciable analgesic effect.

As an opioid-sparing agent

Studies have shown that patients on TCADs have significantly lower morphine requirements. If this is important in a patient's management, or if there are other indications for their use, a TCAD can be prescribed.

UNWANTED EFFECTS

Anticholinergic

These are the most frequent and often the most troublesome side-effects of the TCADs – they may even cause the patient to discontinue the drug. Careful explanation of the likely side-effects and the fact that they may well 'wear off' as the patient develops tolerance will help. The doctor should start with a low initial dose and increase it gradually in order to allow tolerance to develop.

- Dry mouth and drying of all other mucous membranes
- Blurred vision: warn patients about driving and operating heavy machinery, and more mundane tasks such as cooking. It is safer to advise the patient to avoid driving, and similar activities, until the dose is stable and tolerance to unwanted effects has developed
- Increased intraocular pressure
- Urinary retention
- Constipation: this is a particular hazard in people with paraplegia, in whom pseudo-obstruction of the bowel can be precipitated. Constipation is also reported more frequently in children.

There are other anticholinergic reactions which are reported less frequently, for example oesophageal reflux and hyperthermia.

CNS effects

Tricyclics also have a wide variety of unwanted effects on the CNS. Inconvenient and potentially dangerous drowsiness is commonly reported. Sedation is related to blockade of central H_1 histaminergic receptors. Confusion, agitation, nightmares, restlessness and, paradoxically, insomnia also occur.

The tricyclics may even exacerbate underlying psychiatric disorders, including depression, mania and delusional states. They lower the convulsant threshold and fits are not uncommon in susceptible individuals, especially children.

There are also many other possible adverse effects on the CNS which are listed below:

- Fine tremor
- Other extrapyramidal effects, e.g. akathisia, oculogyric crisis, dysarthria
- Dizziness
- Ataxia, incoordination, unsteadiness.

Falls, leading to serious injury, are more common in elderly patients on these drugs. This should be taken into account when prescribing them. If an antidepressant is required a drug with a smaller incidence of drowsiness and blurred vision should be considered.

Cardiovascular effects

A wide variety of unwanted cardiovascular effects have been reported, and it is probably simplest to remember that these drugs are potentially **cardiotoxic** and should be used with extreme caution, if at all, in patients with pre-existing heart disease. Remember that a significant number of people over the age of 50 (and the proportion rises with each decade of life) have silent ischaemic heart disease.

The most important adverse cardiovascular drug reactions are:

- T-wave abnormalities
- conduction disturbances, e.g. bundle branch blocks
- dysrhythmias of all kinds
- syncope and postural hypotension.

Fatal **neuroleptic malignant syndrome** has occurred with TCADs.

Haematological effects

Blood dyscrasias are rare but can be fatal. A white cell and differential count should be performed on any patient who develops fever or other symptoms suggesting neutropenia.

Hepatic effects

It is well known that rises in liver enzymes occur in patients on TCAD therapy. Jaundice and hepatitis have also been reported which have resolved when the drug was stopped. Fatalities have been reported when the drug was continued.

Sensitivity reactions

All types of allergic sensitivity reaction have been recorded. Photosensitivity is known and patients may need to avoid sunlight if this is a problem.

Other adverse effects

Almost every adverse drug reaction has been reported with a TCAD, but patients may develop tolerance to some of the effects if the drug is started at a low dose which is increased slowly.

PRECAUTIONS AND CONTRAINDICATIONS

These largely follow from the adverse drug reactions listed above. If there is a strong contraindication to a TCAD but an antidepressant drug is needed, a newer tricyclic, such as lofepramine, or an SSRI (selective serotonin reuptake inhibitor) should be considered. These drugs do not have the anticholinergic side-effects or α-adrenoceptor blocking activity of a drug such as amitriptyline, nor the effects on noradrenaline reuptake. Evidence to confirm the efficacy of these drugs in pain therapy is not available.

Precautions

Consider the need for a TCAD or the TCAD prescribed:

- in people with a history of urinary retention or prostatic hypertrophy, as urinary retention can be precipitated in susceptible individuals
- in patients with known existing cardiac conduction defects
- in the frail elderly: a wide variety of adverse effects could have damaging consequences, for example sedation contributing to a fall, confusion contributing to a hospital admission in someone previously managing at home
- for patients who must drive, for economic reasons for example, as they are unlikely to stop driving until they have become tolerant to the sedative effects. A newer TCAD or SSRI may be a better choice
- in patients with a family history of the rare neuroleptic malignant syndrome: if this is known it would be an absolute contraindication to the use of these drugs
- in patients with severe depression and a suicide risk: only a small number of tablets should be available to the patient at any one time because of the danger of taking an overdose
- in people with glaucoma.

DRUG INTERACTIONS

A formulary should always be consulted if the patient is taking other drugs, as TCADs interact with a large number of other compounds. The most important are listed below.

- At least 2 weeks should elapse between stopping a TCAD and starting a MAOI.
- At least 2 weeks should elapse between stopping a TCAD and starting an SSRI.
- MAOIs and TCADs should not be prescribed together, although this is sometimes done in the treatment of intractable depression.
- The sedative effect of TCADs will be enhanced by any other sedative drug, including alcohol.
- Cimetidine will decrease the hepatic metabolism of TCADs and so enhance their effects.

Paediatric precautions

These drugs are **not recommended for children** under 16 years old, except in the treatment of nocturnal enuresis. Children are much more susceptible to all the unwanted effects of these drugs.

ADMINISTRATION

Oral

Oral administration of these drugs is the preferred route.

The drugs are long acting and can usually be given once daily, a sedative antidepressant being given at bedtime and a stimulating one in the morning.

Starting dose

Because of genetic differences in the way these drugs are handled by the body there will be a wide variation in the dose needed by different patients to achieve the same effect. The starting dose should be low and increased slowly to achieve a therapeutic effect, but allowing tolerance to the unwanted effects to develop.

Remember:
- *Unwanted* effects start within a few hours.
- *Analgesic* effects start within a few days (2–4).
- *Antidepressant* effects start within a few weeks (4–6).

Stopping the drug

TCADs should not be stopped abruptly as sleep disturbance, irritability and other CNS effects have been reported. Instead, the drug should be tapered off over a period of weeks or months, depending on how long the patient has been taking it.

AMITRIPTYLINE

This is the TCAD which has been most widely used in clinical trials of pain relief and a dose–response curve has been shown for its analgesic action, although there are huge interindividual variations in the plasma level achieved with the same dose. It is a well-established drug and is cheaper than the newer preparations, but there is no doubt that it has a high incidence of unwanted effects, so that some clinicians favour the newer TCADs or one of the SSRIs to avoid these problems. Amitriptyline is a typical TCAD, so the section below includes points that are relevant only to this drug.

ADMINISTRATION

It should normally be given at bedtime, as it is a sedative.

Dosage

As expected, there is a great variation in the doses needed by different patients to achieve the same therapeutic effect, and the dose at which the adverse reactions become intolerable. In a frail elderly patient 10 mg would be an appropriate starting dose and it may not be possible or necessary to increase it further. In a fitter patient 25 mg nocte would be more usual. **Analgesic doses are usually lower than antidepressant doses**. In patients with advanced disease the doses needed both to treat depression and to achieve analgesia are lower, probably because of impaired drug metabolism. Once maximal therapeutic effect is achieved the maintenance dose in depression and chronic non-malignant pain may be lower. Experience has been gained with patients on this drug for many years consecutively.

MIANSERIN

This is related to the tricyclic group of antidepressants: there are no special indications for its use in pain therapy. Agraulocytosis has occurred during treatment with this drug. The manufacturers recommend that monthly monitoring of the white cell count is carried out during the first 3 months of its use, as this is when the problem most frequently arises.

MONOAMINE OXIDASE INHIBITORS

Examples: phenelzine, isocarboxid and trancylpromine.

These should be used cautiously. Their mode of action in pain relief is similar to all antidepressants, outlined at the beginning of this chapter.

They are more hazardous than other antidepressants because of their interactions with tyramine (which is present in many foods) and a number of drugs to produce a dangerous – even fatal – pressor response in the cardiovascular system. They have a specific role in the treatment of **atypical facial pain**, where they are commonly used in combination with a phenothiazine (Motipres).

SELECTIVE SEROTONIN REUPTAKE INHIBITORS

Examples: fluoxetine, fluvoxamine, paroxetine and sertraline.

As their name explains, these drugs selectively block the presynaptic reuptake of serotonin. They are the most recently developed group of antidepressants and are highly selective for serotonin, having a negligible effect on noradrenergic pathways. It is thought that drugs with effects on both serotonergic and monoamine pathways have maximal effect in pain relief, and these drugs are too new for there to be the accumulated clinical experience that there is with the TCADs, but potentiation of opioids and independent analgesic activity has been demonstrated for them. Fluoxetine is used as the model for this section.

PHARMACOKINETICS

Oral absorption

Fluoxetine is well absorbed from the GI tract after oral administration: some 60–80% of the dose is absorbed. The degree of first-pass metabolism is unknown in humans.

Antidepressant effect

Steady-state concentrations of the drug and its metabolite are attained within 2–4 weeks and the antidepressant effect occurs within 1–3 weeks of starting therapy, but its maximal effect will not be seen before 4–6 weeks. The relationship between plasma concentration of the drug and therapeutic effect is not straightforward.

Metabolism

This takes place principally in the liver and a pharmacologically active metabolite, norfluoxetine, is produced. The rate of metabolism is under polygenic control and therefore shows considerable interindividual variations.

The plasma half-lives of fluoxetine and norfluoxetine are considerably prolonged (to an average of 7 and 12 days, respectively) in those with hepatic cirrhosis, but renal disease appears to make little difference to their elimination.

THERAPEUTIC USES IN PAIN RELIEF

These are the same as for the TCADs, i.e. they are used in the management of all types of nerve damage pain. There are far fewer published trials on the use of SSRIs in pain therapy than on TCADs.

Unwanted effects

Because SSRIs are highly selective, increasing only the concentration of serotonin in the CNS, they have far fewer side-effects. Many of their adverse effects are dose related, and outside the normal dose range there is an increase in the severity of unwanted effects without an increase in analgesic efficacy.

CNS effects

The most important symptom is headache, which has been reported in up to one-fifth of patients. Anxiety is not uncommon and appears to be dose related. Other symptoms include drowsiness, fatigue, tremor and dizziness. Insomnia has been reported, but this may also be a symptom of depression and may improve as depression lifts.

Effects on the GI tract

These are the most common adverse effects associated with fluoxetine and include, in descending order of frequency, nausea, diarrhoea, anorexia and dyspepsia. More rarely abdominal pain, changes in taste perception, flatulence and vomiting have been recorded. These and the many other rare symptoms which have been associated with SSRIs may be due to the complex effects that serotonin can have on the gut. If the unwanted effect is not serious and the drug can be continued the patient may become tolerant to it.

Metabolic effects

Weight loss rather than weight gain is associated with fluoxetine because it is an anorectic. It may also change blood glucose concentrations: both hypo- and hyperglycaemia have been reported. Caution is therefore necessary in prescribing this drug to diabetics.

Many other symptoms have been reported in patients taking fluoxetine but they are not definitely associated with the drug. Present evidence suggests that SSRIs do not have major cardiotoxic effects nor important anticholinergic actions, both significant problems with TCADs.

PRECAUTIONS

Fluoxetine and other SSRIs are relatively new drugs, and so clinical experience in patients with concurrent systemic disease or other regular drug therapy is limited. Close monitoring of patients, particularly in these categories, is therefore necessary, especially if any new symptoms or signs develop. Caution is necessary in patients with hepatic or renal impairment or serious cardiovascular disease.

Great care must be given to patients **at risk of suicide** and adequate supervision organized.

Vigilance, with laboratory testing where indicated, is also needed in:

- diabetic patients, because of possible alterations in blood glucose concentrations
- patients who develop skin reactions in the course of treatment with these drugs, as they may herald a serious systemic reaction
- patients with epilepsy, as the convulsant threshold is lowered.

Drug interactions

- The effects of alcohol and all other drugs that act on the CNS can be potentiated.
- There is an increased risk of toxicity if an SSRI is used in conjunction with a MAOI; therefore some weeks (interval depending on the SSRI used) should elapse between the use of these drugs.
- SSRIs interact with all the anticonvulsants and lower the convulsant threshold, so expert advice should be obtained before using them in an epileptic patient.
- SSRIs increase the plasma concentrations of theophylline, selegiline, propranolol and flecainide: the risk of toxicity of these drugs is therefore increased.
- SSRIs should not be prescribed with lithium, as the risk of CNS toxicity is increased.

Stopping SSRIs

Where possible these drugs should be tapered off slowly.

> **Remember, fluoxetine and norfluoxetine have very long half-lives.**

ADMINISTRATION

Oral fluoxetine

This is the route of choice and the drug is usually given once daily (it has a long half-life) in the morning, but if troublesome sedation occurs the dose may be given at bedtime.

The usual dose is 20 mg. Analgesic effects should be apparent before antidepressant ones, but the drug should be continued for 4–6 weeks before deciding that it is not going to help.

THE ANTICONVULSANT DRUGS

The anticonvulsant drugs are a pharmacologically diverse group of compounds which exert their antiepileptic action in three main ways:

- Raising the concentration of inhibitory neurotransmitters (especially γ-aminobutyric acid, GABA).
- Antagonizing excitatory amino acid neurotransmitters
- Inhibition of ion flux across membranes.

Serendipitously they were found also to have an analgesic effect. It has been stated that because of the way in which they affect sodium channels they reduce paroxysmal rather than intermittent neurone firing, but a recent systematic review has suggested that they are equally useful for any pain that has a neuropathic component. It should be remembered that anticonvulsants are not intrinsically analgesic and may not be licensed for this use.

SODIUM VALPROATE

Valproate **increases brain GABA concentrations** both by inhibiting the action of the enzymes that metabolize it and also by increasing its synthesis. Valproate has other actions in the CNS, which may include:

- selectively enhancing the postsynaptic response to GABA in spinal cord neurones
- inhibiting the neuronal uptake of GABA
- a possible effect on the excitatory amino acid aspartate.

PHARMACOKINETICS

Valproate may be given orally or intravenously, but the oral route is preferred. Sodium valproate is converted quickly and almost completely to valproic acid in the stomach, and is then absorbed from the GI tract.

THERAPEUTIC USES IN PAIN THERAPY

Sodium valproate is used in the treatment of neuropathic pain – it is used differently in different centres. Some use it as a first-line drug in this condition; some use it after an antidepressant has been tried, or in combination with an antidepressant. Other authorities recommend it for pain which is stabbing rather than burning, but studies in diabetics show that it can be used in all types of neuropathic pain and a recent systematic review found no difference between anticonvulsants and antidepressants in neuropathic pain.

Unwanted effects

A wide range of unwanted effects have been reported with sodium valproate. The most important include:

- nausea, vomiting and indigestion, which can be minimized if the drug is taken at mealtimes
- sedation and drowsiness
- increased appetite and weight gain
- fatal hepatotoxicity has been reported in some patients on sodium valproate, but those most at risk are children under 2 years of age, on multiple drug therapy and with severe systemic disease
- bleeding disorders from platelet dysfunction
- alopecia, rash and pruritus.

PRECAUTIONS AND CONTRAINDICATIONS

Patients should be warned that their ability to perform complex tasks and operate potentially hazardous machinery will be impaired.

Patients with active liver disease, or with a family history of liver disease, are at greater risk of the dangerous hepatotoxicity that has been reported with valproate. The drug is contraindicated in these groups. In those with a previous history of liver disease and in all children liver function should be closely monitored for the first 6 months of therapy (the 'at risk' period): the drug should be stopped in anyone developing symptoms or signs of liver dysfunction.

As prolonged bleeding is possible with this drug investigation of platelet function is indicated before surgery or invasive procedures.

Pregnancy and lactation

There is an increased risk of neural tube defect with this drug. It may be used in breastfeeding mothers in normal doses.

DRUG INTERACTIONS

- Combinations of anticonvulsants are to be avoided as complex effects on plasma concentrations are produced. There is no place for them in pain therapy.
- Alcohol and all CNS depressants will increase these effects produced by sodium valproate.
- The pharmacological effects of antidepressant drugs, particularly MAOIs, are increased by sodium valproate and the dose may need to be decreased.
- As bleeding disorders are associated with valproate extra care should be used in patients taking drugs such as aspirin or warfarin, which affect coagulation.

DOSAGE AND ADMINISTRATION

Valproate should be taken by mouth, and may be given at mealtimes to avoid gastric irritation. It is often given in divided doses two or three times a day, but it is long acting and a single night-time dose may be more convenient. A 6-week trial is necessary before its therapeutic usefulness can be assessed. Most patients benefit from 600 mg daily, but an elderly or frail person may only require 200 mg and sometimes it is necessary to give 1 g. It is best to start with a low dose and increase this slowly to avoid problems with sedation.

CARBAMAZEPINE

Carbamazepine was first used in trigeminal neuralgia. It has structural similarities to the tricyclic antidepressants. Pharmacologically it is similar to phenytoin: its anticonvulsant properties are due to the suppression of post-tetanic potentiation of monosynaptic reflexes, and it also depresses post-tetanic potentiation at the neuromuscular junction. The pain of trigeminal neuralgia is helped by the reduction of synaptic transmission in the trigeminal nucleus. Carbamazepine is used in the same way as sodium valproate in the treatment of all types of neuropathic pain.

PHARMACOKINETICS

Absorption

Carbamazepine is absorbed only slowly from the GI tract, and after oral administration peak plasma concentrations are reached in 2–8 hours. It may take 4 days to reach steady-state plasma concentrations. Therapeutic plasma concentrations are quoted as 4–12 mg/1 (20–50 μmol/l) for both trigeminal neuralgia and the control of epilepsy. The plasma concentrations reached after the same dose of drug in different patients varies considerably. Autoinduction of metabolic enzymes takes place and the dose needs to be increased after 1–2 weeks.

THERAPEUTIC USES IN PAIN RELIEF

Trigeminal neuralgia

Nearly all patients with trigeminal neuralgia will respond to carbamazepine, at least initially. Failure of response is said to be diagnostic.

Other types of neuropathic pain

Like sodium valproate, carbamazepine can be effective in treating all kinds of neuropathic pain of both malignant and non-malignant origin.

UNWANTED EFFECTS

These can be minimized by using a small initial dose (100 mg b.d.) and increasing it by weekly increments of 100 mg b.d. until the maximum dose or the desired pharmacological effect is reached.

CNS

Dizziness, drowsiness and ataxia can all be troublesome, especially in elderly patients. Other CNS side-effects include confusion, headache, nystagmus and speech disturbances.

The GI tract

Carbamazepine causes nausea, vomiting, abdominal pain and constipation. The gastric irritation can be minimized by taking it with food.

Cardiovascular effects

Carbamazepine can have extremely dangerous toxic effects on the CVS – it is contraindicated for patients with atrioventricular conduction defects. It can exacerbate all forms of cardiac disease.

Haematological effects

Leucopenia has been reported and, more rarely, aplastic anaemia.

Hepatic effects

Abnormalities of liver function, of all types, have been reported.

Other unwanted effects

There is a wide range of adverse effects associated with carbamazepine therapy. The most important have been mentioned above, but it is important to reassess therapy if the patient devlops a new symptom while taking carbamazepine.

Other conditions in which carbamazepine should be used with great caution, if at all, include:

- liver disease
- renal impairment.

All patients receiving carbamazepine should have baseline FBC (full blood count) and LFTs (liver function tests) carried out, and periodic monitoring while taking the drug. Carbamazepine should be stopped if abnormalities develop.

It is necessary to warn patients starting therapy that their ability to perform complex tasks or operate machinery will be impaired, at least in the early days.

CONTRAINDICATIONS

- AV conduction defects
- A history of sensitivity to the tricyclics
- A history of bone marrow suppression, or a haematological reaction to another drug
- Porphyria.

Pregnancy and lactation

There is an increased incidence of neural tube defects in the infants of women taking carbamazepine. Its use for pain therapy is not advisable in women who are, or may become, pregnant, nor those who are breastfeeding.

Drug interactions

Many drug interactions are possible and physicians prescribing carbamazepine should refer to a formulary for advice. The most important interactions are:

- with many other anticonvulsants
- an increase in carbamazepine levels with verapamil
- an increase in plasma carbamazepine with erythromycin
- increased rate of metabolism of warfarin: monitor blood clotting function
- a decrease in the efficacy of the oral contraceptive pill.

DOSAGE AND ADMINISTRATION

Oral

This is the preferred route: the drug should be taken with meals to decrease the likelihood of gastric irritation.

The starting dose of carbamazepine should be low and increased slowly to minimize the risk of adverse effects and toxicity. In the treatment of pain the quoted therapeutic range for carbamazepine can be used as a guide, but the drug should not be abandoned until it has been given for at least 6 weeks. (see Management of Neuropathic Pain, Chapter 19).

Lamotrigine is chemically unrelated to other anticonvulsants. It may find a place in pain therapy as it inhibits the release of the principal fast excitatory neurotransmitter glutamate, which is involved in nociception. It has few side-effects, a long half-life and few drug interactions.

Phenytoin was the anticonvulsant most used in pain therapy until it was superseded by carbamazepine (which is pharmacologically very similar) and sodium valproate. It may still be prescribed where other therapies have failed. Its drawbacks include its narrow therapeutic window, many drug interactions and important unwanted effects.

Clonazepam is a benzodiazepine which is useful in the management of both epilepsy and neuropathic pain. Benzodiazepines are addictive and should be avoided in chronic pain states where possible.

CHAPTER 7

MISCELLANEOUS DRUGS USED IN PAIN CONTROL

In this section drugs which do not fit into other categories and those which are used only rarely are briefly considered. Incontrovertible evidence is not available for many pain-relieving treatments, though much is being uncovered by systematic reviews, but many of the drugs mentioned here are still experimental or have been given to only a small number of patients. Some are administered only after other drugs and strategies have been tried.

CORTICOSTEROIDS

Corticosteroids (often shortened to steroids) are hormones secreted by the adrenal cortex or their synthetic analogues. Their pharmacological actions are very complex and wide ranging, affecting nearly all body systems. They cannot be classed as analgesics in their own right, but they are **co-analgesics**, i.e. they are given largely to enhance the effects of drugs with a proven direct analgesic effect, such as morphine. It is likely that their most important pain-relieving property is their anti-inflammatory effect, and they are most often used in the pain of advanced cancer as their unwanted effects, when they are used over a long period of time, can be very serious.

This section is not exhaustive. Corticosteroids are used in nearly all branches of medicine and given by nearly all routes of administration, including injection into joints and soft-tissue injuries. Only dexamethasone and prednisolone will be considered in any detail, as these are the preparations most commonly used in pain therapy.

DEXAMETHASONE

This is a synthetic glucocorticoid with only minor mineralocorticoid activity but powerful anti-inflammatory effects. It is very potent, and this reduces the number of tablets needed to achieve a significant effect.

PHARMACOKINETICS

Dexamethasone sodium phosphate is well absorbed by mouth and by inhalation, but it is also given parenterally and less frequently by injection into soft-tissue lesions, into joints and into the synovium. Triamcinolone, which has a very long duration of action, is more commonly used for this indication.

Half-life

The length of time that a corticosteroid suppresses the hypothalamopituitary axis (HPA) is called its **biological half-life**, and this is more important in clinical practice than its plasma half-life. The biological half-life of dexamethasone is 2–3 days.

THERAPEUTIC USES IN PAIN RELIEF

It is thought that dexamethasone may help cancer pain by reducing the oedema that surrounds a tumour. Tumour mass is reduced and thereby pressure on surrounding structures, including nerves. The analgesic effect is greatest in a confined space, and dexamethasone is used for:

- the headache associated with raised intracranial pressure from cerebral tumours
- nerve compression pain, often in conjunction with an opioid/antidepressant
- malignant bone pain

In non-malignant pain dexamethasone is used for:

- chronic back pain, when it is given in combination with a local anaesthetic into the epidural space (unlicensed indication)
- the management of acutely inflamed joints, where it may be injected into the affected area

Unwanted effects

These are legion and can be very damaging, especially when corticosteroids are used over a long period of time.

> **Corticosteroids should always be used at the lowest possible dose for the shortest possible time.**

Short-term use (less than 2 weeks) is unlikely to produce significant adverse effects, but in the longer term (and the definition of this depends on the patient and the dose administered) adrenocortical insufficiency will occur, so that a patient on long-term dexamethasone will require an increased dose when subjected to stresses such as trauma, surgery, acute illness etc.

> **No patient on chronic corticosteroid therapy should have their drug withdrawn suddenly, as fatal acute adrenal insufficiency can follow.**

Corticosteroids can cause a wide range of problems, including muscle wasting, osteoporosis and avascular necrosis of the femoral head, and in the susceptible individual these can come on within a few weeks. Often the most distressing to the patient are the signs of Cushing's syndrome – moon face, abdominal striae and weight gain with central fat deposition – which may appear within a few days of starting the drug. Sleep disturbance and a feeling of restlessness may start within 24 hours.

A more complete list will be found in standard textbooks of therapeutics, but in pain relief corticosteroids are most frequently prescribed to patients with advanced cancer, where the benefits of careful, thoughtful prescribing should outweigh the risks.

CONTRAINDICATIONS

- Known hypersensitivity to glucocorticoids
- In patients with active viral or bacterial illness (or previous history of TB), unless there is an overwhelming indication
- In patients with active peptic ulceration
- In patients with osteoporosis, except where there is an overwhelming indication
- In patients with a recent myocardial infarction, as ventricular wall rupture has been reported

PRECAUTIONS

Before prescribing a corticosteroid ensure that it is really necessary, and explain the unwanted effects to the patient and why it is needed in his or her case. Ensure that the patient understands that:

- she or he must report early to the doctor if an intercurrent infection develops and that a temporary increase in dose may be necessary
- he or she must not stop taking the drug suddenly
- the reduction of steroid dosage, even when very slow, is associated with a number of symptoms (headache, pyrexia, myalgia), often called 'steroid pseudorheumatism'
- if she or he is not immune to chicken pox and is exposed while on steroids, passive immunization must be given as soon as possible, as this is a very dangerous illness in the immunosuppressed.

Dexamethasone, and other corticosteroids, should be used with caution in patients on NSAIDs, as there is evidence that these increase the risk of peptic ulceration. Patients with cirrhosis will often require a lower than anticipated dose of dexamethasone. Patients with a psychotic illness may be more susceptible to the neuropsychiatric complications of steroid therapy. Diabetes may develop or be exacerbated while someone is taking corticosteroids.

Paediatric prescribing

This is for specialists only. Children with advanced cancer seem to receive less benefit and suffer more unwanted effects from steroid therapy for the treatment of raised intracranial pressure, for example, and other analgesic drugs need to be tried to their maximum extent before a steroid is used.

DRUG INTERACTIONS

- Patients taking drugs that induce hepatic microsomal enzymes – and this includes many anticonvulsants – may require increased doses of dexamethasone.
- The risk of peptic ulceration is increased if a patient takes a steroid and an NSAID simultaneously.
- Dexamethasone increases potassium loss, and this will be enhanced by any other drugs with the same effect (thiazide diuretics, for example).
- The antibody response to vaccination will be reduced and live vaccines may be hazardous.

ADMINISTRATION

Oral

This is the route of first choice in the treatment of cancer pain. It is preferable to give it as a single morning dose, since if it is taken later in the day it may cause or exacerbate insomnia. There is no evidence that giving it as alternate-day therapy significantly reduces its unwanted effects.

Starting dose

This depends on the condition being treated. Generally in the treatment of raised intracranial pressure the starting dose will be 8–12 mg once daily (sometimes higher in patients taking anticonvulsants), reducing after 3–5 days (by which time maximum therapeutic effect will have been seen) until the lowest effective dose is attained. Clinical signs are used as a measure of effectiveness: for example the resolution of neurological symptoms, including hemiplegia or headache.

Introduction of dexamethasone into a lesion, joint or the synovium

It is always preferable to use steroids locally rather than systemically, as there will be a lower incidence of unwanted effects. Triamcinolone is most commonly used for injection into joints.

Epidural

Dexamethasone is sometimes combined with bupivacaine for intermittent epidural injection to ameliorate chronic back pain (see Chapter 16). This is an unlicensed indication and should only be carried out by a specialist in chronic pain therapy: evidence is conflicting about its efficacy and, indeed, whether it **causes** neurological damage.

PREDNISOLONE

This is a synthetic corticosteroid and, like dexamethasone, it has minimal mineralocorticoid activity. Prednisolone has many similarities to dexamethasone but differs in three important respects:

- Its biological half-life is shorter: it produces suppression of the HPA for 18–36 hours
- Its plasma half-life is shorter: 3–4 hours rather than 5–6 hours
- It is less potent than dexamethasone: 1 mg dexamethasone has the same pharmacological activity as 7.5 mg of prednisolone, so that 30 mg prednisolone is equivalent to 4 mg dexamethasone.

For the rest of its clinical pharmacology in pain relief, see Dexamethasone.

CAPSAICIN

This is a naturally occurring alkaloid which can be extracted from chilli peppers. It affects the synthesis, storage, transport and release of substance P in nociceptive fibres. When applied topically it will cause degeneration of nociceptive C fibres.

It has been developed as a cream (0.075%) for the treatment of postherpetic neuralgia (and other neuropathic pains) and is applied topically to affected areas five times daily. Its only important adverse effect seems to be a burning or tingling when first applied. This lessens with continued treatment (it is intolerable for only a few patients). It is thought that application of capsaicin causes a release of substance P from C fibres, which become depleted of this substance with repeated use of the cream. This depletion results in reduced pain transmission. When capsaicin application ceases substance P will return to its former levels.

CLONIDINE

This is a centrally acting mixed α_1- and α_2-adrenoceptor agonist, with α_2 activity predominating. Its inhibition of sympathetic vasomotor centres, in the medulla oblongata, causes reduced peripheral sympathetic nervous activity. Its analgesic action, which has been demonstrated in humans, is not fully understood but is likely to result from **modification of central and peripheral neurotransmitter activity**. Its unwanted effects include hypotension, bradycardia, dry mouth and sedation. It is used intraspinally, in conjunction with morphine and local anaesthetics, to treat cancer-related neuropathic pain. Clonidine is useful as single agent in only a minority of patients. It has also been found to prolong the effect of local anaesthetic caudals used for perioperative analgesia in paediatric surgery. A transdermal preparation is available and has been used in the treatment of diabetic neuropathy, with mixed results.

THE BISPHOSPHONATES

Examples: disodium etidronate, disodium pamidronate, sodium clodronate and alendronate. Bisphosphonates **inhibit bone resorption** by their effects on osteoclasts. One of their primary uses is in the treatment of the hypercalcaemia of malignancy. It is thought that hypercalcaemia can precipitate or exacerbate pain from bony metastases, but the primary treatment of bone pain remains radiotherapy, NSAIDs and opioids.

Other uses:

- Treatment of Paget's disease
- Treatment of osteoporosis
- Prevention/treatment of skeletal-related morbidity in bony metastases from cancer and multiple myeloma (for example pathological fractures, spinal cord compression).

ADMINISTRATION

Bisphosphonates are poorly absorbed by mouth (0.5–2.0% of an administered dose, even on an empty stomach) and they are usually given by intermittent intravenous injection for the treatment of hypercalcaemia and bone pain. (They are used orally in the treatment of osteoporosis.) In some centres this may be followed up by much larger doses of oral therapy, and in others clinical and biochemical markers are followed and further intravenous therapy given when required.

Disodium pamidronate and sodium clodronate are the most commonly used drugs in the hypercalcaemia and bone pain associated with malignancy. There have been reports of clodronate being usefully administered subcutaneously (it is not licensed for this route). The aminophosphonates (pamidronate, for example) have greater potency but also a higher incidence of unwanted effects, and have caused intolerable local irritation when given subcutaneously.

Unwanted effects

Oral therapy

These drugs have to be given on an empty stomach and cause nausea, vomiting, diarrhoea and abdominal pain.

Intravenous therapy only

Thrombophlebitis (especially with rapid injection), hypocalcaemia, urticaria and angio-oedema.

CONTRAINDICATIONS

Renal impairment, pregnancy and lactation.

Disodium pamidronate

By slow intravenous infusion – 15–60 mg according to plasma calcium level (maximum 90 mg as one dose). There is no oral preparation.

Sodium clodronate

By slow intravenous infusion – 300 mg daily for maximum 7–10 days, or by single-dose infusion of 1.5 g
By mouth: 1.6–3.2 g daily in divided doses.

KETAMINE

Ketamine was developed as an anaesthetic; it induces a state called **dissociative anaesthesia** in which the patient's eyes are open and they may appear awake but are unaware of their surroundings; there is profound analgesia. While emerging from this state many patients experience vivid dreams, unpleasant illusions and flashback phenomena, and for this reason ketamine is now rarely used in the UK as an adult anaesthetic agent. At lower doses it can produce analgesia without affecting conscious level and without causing emergence phenomena.

Ketamine has now found a place in neuropathic pain management, particularly in cancer patients and in combination with morphine. Its analgesic effects are thought to stem from its actions as an **NMDA antagonist** (see Chapter 1). It is not a first-line agent and should be used after advice from a pain specialist or palliative care physician.

PHARMACOKINETICS

Ketamine is most commonly administered by the i.v. and i.m. routes, but has been used orally, rectally, intraspinally and intranasally.

When used parenterally bioavailability is greater than 90%. Although ketamine is well absorbed by the oral route it is subject to extensive first-pass metabolism and its bioavailability is very unpredictable – figures of 10–20% are quoted.

Plasma half-life is between 150 and 240 minutes.

Peak analgesia occurs:

- within 15–30 minutes when used by the intramuscular route
- within 30–60 minutes when used by the oral route.

Analgesia lasts about 3 hours.

Metabolism

This takes place principally in the liver, where the drug is *n*-demethylated to norketamine before further biotransformation takes place. **Norketamine** is pharmacologically active, having one-third the analgesic potency of its parent and also exerting hypnotic effects. It is thought that the high serum level of norketamine produced by first-pass metabolism in oral administration may help to explain why oral ketamine has been reported in some studies to produce comparable analgesia at lower plasma concentrations than with parenteral use. Ketamine may safely be used in patients with renal impairment.

THERAPEUTIC USES IN PAIN RELIEF

Ketamine is used for:

- analgesia for short procedures, such as changing burns dressings
- as a second-line drug for the treatment of neuropathic pain, particularly in cancer patients
- battlefield analgesia: its cardiovascular effects are particularly useful here.

UNWANTED EFFECTS

Nervous system

Used alone, particularly in adults, ketamine produces a frightening floating sensation and unpleasant flashback phenomena. These can be reduced by warning patients about their incidence beforehand and the use of benzodiazepines as part of the premedication technique.

Ketamine is a CNS stimulant, producing a rise in cerebral metabolism, cerebral blood flow and intracranial pressure.

Cardiovascular system

A single intravenous dose of ketamine will produce a transient, significant rise in the heart rate and blood pressure which may last for 5 minutes. Dysrhythmias are rare. These effects are not important when ketamine is used as an infusion.

PRECAUTIONS

Ketamine should be used with caution, if at all, in the following groups:

- Patients with hypertensive disease
- Patients with raised intracranial pressure
- Patients with glaucoma
- Patients with psychiatric illness.

Pregnancy and lactation

Ketamine causes an increase in uterine tone, crosses the placenta and may cause fetal depression. It should especially be avoided in hypertensive pregnant patients.

ADMINISTRATION IN PAIN RELIEF

Ketamine is generally used as a subcutaneous infusion when used to treat neuropathic cancer pain. When used orally the parenteral preparation is given but disguised, as it is unacceptably bitter for most patients.

Suggested subcutaneous dosages: 0.05–0.10 mg/kg stat over 5 minutes followed by an infusion of 0.05–0.10 mg/kg/h.

BACLOFEN

γ-amino butyric acid (GABA) is an inhibitory neurotransmitter and baclofen is a **GABA agonist** which acts both at spinal cord level and centrally. It is used orally and intraspinally in the treatment of painful contractures and spasms resulting from chronic neurological diseases such as multiple sclerosis and motor neurone disease. Its most important adverse effects are sedation and hypotonia: these may be avoided if any necessary dose increases are slow.

CLASS I ANTIDYSRHYTHMICS

Examples: mexiletine, flecainide, lignocaine.

All these drugs have membrane-stabilizing activity, which is why they are useful as antidysrhythmic agents. Apart from its local anaesthetic activity (see Chapter 4) i.v. lignocaine is known to have some analgesic effects, but it cannot be used orally. Mexiletine and flecainide are used in the treatment of neuropathic pain, particularly in cancer patients but also in those suffering from diabetic neuropathy. Mexiletine has been reported to be effective in dysaesthesias associated with multiple sclerosis. Both can be taken by mouth, and a much smaller dose is used than in the management of dysrhythmias. Flecainide is no longer favoured by cardiologists since a large multicentre study demonstrated an excess of sudden deaths in those patients treated with it following myocardial infarction: this problem has not so far been reported in cancer patients. Some authorities advise that other potentially cardiotoxic drugs, such as tricyclics, should not be used concurrently, and that there should be a washout period between a tricyclic finishing and flecainide being started.

MIDAZOLAM

This is a short-acting benzodiazepine. It is the most lipid soluble of its class, having twice the affinity of diazepam for the benzodiazepine receptor. It is dispensed as a water-soluble pharmacologically inactive form with a closed imidazole ring, so that it is water-soluble and easily given parenterally. When it enters the patient the ring opens at the higher body pH and it becomes lipid soluble, crossing easily into the CNS.

Midazolam is used in pain therapy:

- intraspinally to enhance antinociception produced by opioids by increasing the affinity of the opioid receptor for opioid agonist
- as a coanalgesic in cancer pain, when it may be given subcutaneously, intravenously or intrathecally to reduce anxiety and possibly to enhance opioid-induced analgesia.

METHOTRIMEPRAZINE

This is a phenothiazine which has demonstrated analgesic activity – 20 mg i.m. is as potent as 10 mg of i.m. morphine, and lasts for about 3 hours. It is very sedating (and is often specifically used for this purpose in the terminally ill patient) and its α-adrenoceptor blocking action causes postural hypotension. It may be useful in combination with other analgesics or as part of a symptom control regimen for administration in a syringe driver. Its analgesic activity is thought to be due to its actions as an NMDA antagonist (see Chapter 1), but it is almost never used purely for analgesia.

CALCITONIN

Salmon calcitonin is a polypeptide hormone which binds to osteoclast receptors and inhibits their activity. Its possible specific analgesic effects were first noticed in animal studies, and it has been used to treat the pain of **metastatic bone disease** when other drugs have failed. It is also used in the management of phantom limb pain. It may be given by i.m. or i.v. injection or taken intranasally.

CHAPTER 8

NEUROSTIMULATION

TRANSCUTANEOUS NERVE STIMULATION (TENS)

INTRODUCTION

Electrical stimulation for the relief of pain has been used since ancient times, but its modern use dates from the late 1960s following publication of the Gate Theory of Pain. TENS was used to predict the likely success of spinal cord stimulation, but was found to be therapeutic per se.

MODE OF ACTION

Stimulation of large-diameter afferent fibres activates (segmental) inhibitory processes in the dorsal horn of the spinal cord. The precise mechanism of this is unknown, but probably involves both pre- and postsynaptic inhibitory mechanisms. The role of endogenous opioids in this inhibition is unclear, since naloxone fails to block the effect of high-frequency TENS. Activation of descending inhibitory mechanisms may contribute to the analgesic effect.

In common with other pain-relieving therapies there is a placebo component to TENS, although this rapidly declines after starting therapy.

INDICATIONS

The use of TENS has been described in almost every painful condition.

Acute pain

- **Postoperative pain**: Open studies have shown efficacy following abdominal, thoracic, orthopaedic and obstetric procedures, although some randomized double-blind controlled trials have shown no greater effect than placebo.
- **Labour pain**: Used widely in the early stages of labour. Electrodes usually placed at T10–L1.
- **Angina**: Successful use has been described. Reduces ST segment depression, increases working capacity and increases tolerance to pacing.

Chronic pain

Conditions for which TENS may be useful:

- Neuropathic pain
  - postherpetic neuralgia
  - phantom limb pain
  - stump pain
  - peripheral nerve injury
  - Complex Regional Pain Syndrome (CRPS)

- Low back pain (including nerve root pain)
- Musculoskeletal pain
- Facial pain
  - trigeminal neuralgia
  - atypical facial pain
- Pain associated with malignant disease.

CONTRAINDICATIONS

These are few but important:

- Stimulation of the pregnant uterus. There are very few data available on the effects on pregnancy, and it is safest to avoid its use, especially in the first trimester. TENS should probably be restricted to pain relief in labour.
- Presence of a cardiac pacemaker. May be hazardous, particularly to demand pacemakers. May be safer for fixed-rate pacemakers but should be discussed with a cardiologist. (Use of TENS should also be avoided in the presence of other electronic implanted devices.)
- Stimulation over the anterior neck. May stimulate the carotid sinus or the nerves to the laryngeal muscles.

PRACTICAL ISSUES

Patient selection

It is difficult to predict who will be helped by TENS, but patients must be willing and able to use the device.

Equipment

TENS equipment comprises a stimulator connected via leads to electrodes which are applied to the patient's skin (Figure 8.1). Large numbers of stimulators are available, but in their most basic form feature:

- combined on/off/amplitude control 0–50 mA
- frequency control 0–100 Hz

  Useful additional features include:
- ability to change mode, e.g. from continuous to pulsed
- pulse width control 0.1–0.5 ms (increasing pulse width reduces the current required for excitation).

Electrodes are usually made of carbon rubber and are applied to the skin with conductive jelly and fixed with tape: Self-adhesive electrodes are available.

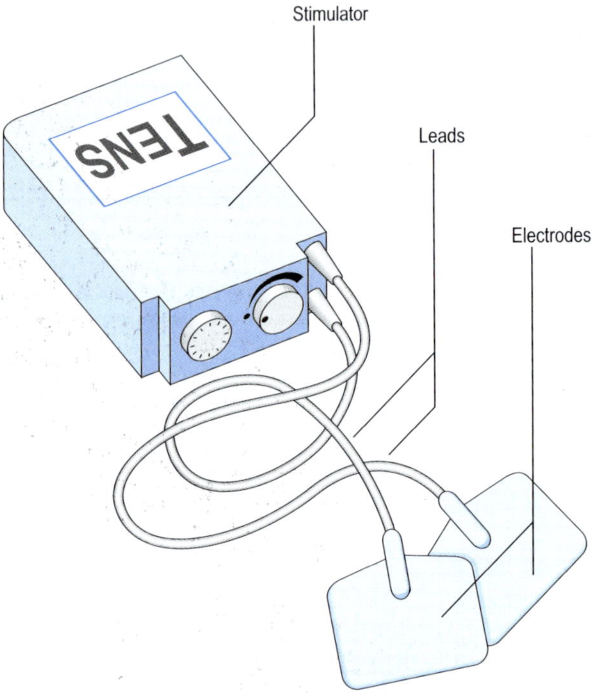

Fig. 8.1 TENS apparatus.

Positioning electrodes

It may take some time to find the optimal site for each patient and they should be encouraged to experiment. Where possible, electrodes should be placed over the painful site or over nerves innervating the painful area. Limb electrodes should be placed longitudinally, and on the trunk in the axis of the dermatome. Electrodes are placed in pairs, usually 1–2 cm apart. Large areas may need more than one pair of electrodes: this can be achieved with a dual-channel stimulator or a double adaptor lead.

Modes of stimulation are summarized in Table 8.1

Trial of TENS should last for at least 1 hour but often needs to be much longer. Preferably patients should take the equipment home, since pain relief may increase over several weeks. Patients should be advised to use the device

TABLE 8.1 TENS: common modes of stimulation

Mode	*Stimulation characteristics*
Conventional TENS	Frequency 30–150 Hz (most patients prefer 40–70 Hz) Low-intensity 10–30 mA (patients should adjust amplitude to the maximum comfortable level – the sensation should not be painful)
Burst (pulsed) TENS	Trains of high frequency (bursts of 100 Hz at 1–2 Hz) Low-intensity 10–30 mA
Acupuncture-like TENS	Bursts of 100 Hz at 1–2 Hz High-intensity 20–50 mA May be useful for those not responding to conventional TENS. More uncomfortable for patient. Partially reversed by naloxone, so probably different mode of action from conventional TENS

for up to 3 hours thrice daily initially, but should be encouraged to use it for as long as necessary to give adequate pain relief. Some patients may experience a period of poststimulation analgesia lasting minutes to hours.

Tolerance

This may occur months after starting TENS therapy. It may be the result of diminished neurotransmitter release or downregulation of receptors. It may be overcome by changing the pulse pattern or by the use of more sophisticated devices which generate random pulse output or multielectrode devices to which pulses are randomly distributed. TENS may be withdrawn for a period and then reinstituted.

Safety

TENS is usually a safe method of analgesia compared to pain-relieving medications and interventional therapies. Skin irritation can usually be avoided by attention to hygiene, careful cleaning of electrodes and changing electrode site every 24 hours. Allergy to electrodes, jelly or tape can be resolved by using an alternative product.

Efficacy

There are widely variable figures published for the efficacy of TENS, and it is difficult to conduct properly controlled trials. However, the results of conventional studies suggest that TENS should be considered a safe and useful first-line therapy for many painful conditions.

SPINAL CORD STIMULATION

INTRODUCTION

Spinal cord stimulation (SCS) was introduced for the control of pain in 1967 and, as with TENS, was a clinical application of the Gate Control Theory of Pain, the intention being to inhibit C-fibre activity by stimulating Aβ fibres in the dorsal columns of the spinal cord. Since that time it has been used for a wide variety of other indications, including angina, peripheral vascular disease and motor disorders.

MODE OF ACTION

It is not clear precisely how spinal cord stimulation works. Stimulation of the dorsal columns is important for the technique to be effective (hence, it is often known as Dorsal Column Stimulation (DCS)), but other pathways, such as the corticospinal and sympathetic pathways, are also stimulated. Stimulation may cause segmental suppression of nociceptive transmission or may electrically interfere with ascending and descending polysynaptic reflexes. Work with both animals and humans has elucidated possible neurohumoral mechanisms for its analgesic actions. Increases in serotonin metabolites and substance P (which is thought to have an inhibitory role in nociceptive transmission in the dorsal horn) result from SCS.

INDICATIONS

SCS has been used in a variety of conditions with variable success. The technique seems to be most useful in pain of neuropathic origin (see Box), particularly in the presence of autonomic disturbance. It is being increasingly used in the management of angina pectoris and peripheral vascular disease.

Neuropathic pain conditions for which SCS may be useful

Phantom limb pain
Complex Regional Pain Syndrome
Failed back surgery with neurological damage
Plexus avulsions
Peripheral nerve lesions

Predictive factors for success have remained elusive but the importance of psychological screening has been emphasized in most published case series. Response to TENS is a poor predictor for success with SCS.

PRACTICAL ISSUES

Early stimulators used plate electrodes placed directly over the dorsal columns in a surgical procedure. Percutaneous electrodes placed using X-ray screening are now much more frequently used.

Trial stimulation

It is agreed that success rates for the implantation of permanent stimulators is markedly increased by prior insertion of a temporary electrode epidurally, producing stimulation in the region of reported pain. The temporary electrode is left in place for a week, during which time the patient experiments with different stimulus parameters (pulse width, frequency, intensity) for most effective pain relief. Only those with greater than 75% pain relief should go on to have permanent electrode insertion.

Permanent electrodes

These may be unipolar, bipolar or multipolar (multipolar is preferred). They may be inserted at laminectomy under general anaesthetic, or preferably percutaneously with the patient awake. The electrodes may be attached to a subcutaneously implanted receiver activated by a radiofrequency device in an external stimulator. Alternatively, wholly intracorporeal systems which can be externally programmed are available. Optimum siting of the electrode should be used to produce paraesthesia over the whole painful area, but usually cervical implantation is most useful for upper limb and trunk pain, and mid-thoracic placement for lower limb pain.

COMPLICATIONS

These are summarized in Table 8.2.

TABLE 8.2 Complications of spinal cord stimulation

Complication	*Comment*
Infection	
Bacterial	May be minimized by good surgical technique. Treated by removal of stimulator and antibiotic therapy
Aseptic meningitis	
Technical failures	Reported as high as 70% in some series.
Electrode migration	Commoner with percutaneous route.
Wire breakage	Better wire exit angle with open procedure
Fibrotic changes around stimulation tip of electrode	
Radicular dysaesthesia	Results from excessively paramedian placement of electrode

OUTCOME

Firm outcome data are hard to find because of the difficulty of performing blind randomized controlled trials in patients. Many case series contain rather heterogeneous diagnostic groups, which makes outcome in a given condition difficult to assess. Several case series have been published for patients following failed back surgery, which show about 50% long-term pain relief.

CONCLUSION

SCS may provide effective, safe pain relief in carefully selected patients. It is a costly procedure, and more data are needed to determine which type of patient this therapy will help.

DEEP BRAIN STIMULATION

Stimulation of the brain for pain control was first used in the early 1960s and is now an accepted technique for the relief of a number of chronic painful conditions refractory to conventional treatment. The commonest sites for stimulation are:

- in the caudal medial thalamic area around the third ventricle (periventricular grey, PVG) and at the junction of the third ventricle and aqueduct of Sylvius (periaqueductal grey, PAG)
- in somatosensory areas of the ventrobasal thalamus, particularly the ventroposterior lateral (VPL) and ventroposterior medial (VPM) nuclei
- in the motor cortex for thalamic pain (see Chapter 1).

The mechanism of action is unknown but is probably related to stimulation of descending inhibitory pathways originating in the midbrain, extending through the reticular formation and travelling from the medulla via dorsolateral tracts to the dorsal horn of the spinal cord. The role of endogenous opioid mechanisms is unclear. NMDA may play a role.

It was originally said that PAG/PVG stimulation was most appropriate for nociceptive (non-neuropathic) pain, whereas VPM/VPL stimulation was more appropriate for neurogenic-type pain. Numerous clinical examples do not obey this 'rule' and clinical pain syndromes often have both nociceptive and neuropathic elements. Selection of patients should be based on:

- well defined aetiology
- pain severely disruptive of life
- absence of major psychological problems
- other attempts at pain management unsuccessful and spontaneous resolution excluded.

Target localization is usually achieved with magnetic resonance scanning and electrodes are implanted stereotactically under local anaesthesia. Stimulation of the PAG/PVG may be accompanied by sensations of warmth, wellbeing and immediate pain relief. Unpleasant sensations such as nervousness, anxiety, sense of impending doom and agitation probably represent less accurate target localization. Stimulation of VPL/VPM nuclei usually evokes paraesthesiae only (rarely muscular contractions at higher stimulus amplitudes).

A successful period of trial stimulation is followed by internalization of electrodes under general anaesthesia.

There are few well controlled studies of the efficacy of deep brain stimulation – measurements of outcome vary widely and the results are not analysed with enough rigour to demontrate significance. Reported success rates vary from 14 to 100%. Similarly the precise complication rate is unknown, but is probably in the region of 20%. Problems usually relate to direct neuronal injury caused by electrode insertion, related intracranial haemorrhage or hardware dysfunction such as electrode breakage or infection. Not all complications are permanent, but persisting neurological deficit and death have been reported.

Success is most likely to be achieved with a team approach, involving neurosurgeons experienced in stereotactic surgery, pain clinicians and psychologists. Deep brain stimulation is a highly invasive and expensive technique and should probably be reserved for those with severely incapacitating pain in whom all other therapies have failed.

ACUPUNCTURE

INTRODUCTION

Western interest in the ancient Chinese practice of acupuncture has increased over the past few decades, and there is an increasing understanding of the mechanisms of action that underly its pain-relieving effect. The procedure involves the insertion of fine needles through selected skin points. The needles are then 'stimulated' manually or electrically to provide a high-intensity low-frequency stimulus to the patient. Different methods of acupuncture exist, with variations in acupuncture point selection and the nature and duration of stimulation. The practice has been used (successfully) to treat a huge range of aetiologically diverse medical conditions and pain states.

MODE OF ACTION

A number of clinical observations suggest that intact afferent transmission is needed for acupuncture to be effective. The technique does not work if:

- acupuncture points are infiltrated with local anaesthetic prior to stimulation
- a stimulus is applied below the level of the block in a patient undergoing subarachnoid (spinal) anaesthesia
- the stimulus is applied to a distant site in a patient with hemiplegia or other pathological deafferentation state.

The responses of dorsal horn neurones to noxious stimuli can be powerfully inhibited by activation of Aδ fibres. This segmental effect is probably mediated by enkephalinergic interneurones in laminae I and II of the dorsal horn. Activation of descending (serotonergic) neurones from the brainstem also excite these inhibitory enkephalinergic interneurones, and this probably forms the basis of heterosegmental acupuncture.

It has also been observed in both animals and man that nociceptive transmission in some neurones can be inhibited by noxious stimulation (of any type – thermal, chemical, mechanical etc.) remote from the receptive fields of those neurones. This has been described as diffuse noxious inhibitory control (DNIC). These effects are enhanced by precursors of serotonin and are diminished by serotonin antagonists and naloxone, which emphasizes the role of serotonin and endogenous opioids in the acupuncture analgesia effect.

Traditional acupuncture points are similar to trigger points and are mostly closely related to the course of underlying peripheral nerves. It has been suggested that they represent loci at which bundles of Aδ afferents and sympathetic efferents penetrate superficial fascia and muscle.

EFFICACY AND SIDE-EFFECTS

There are few double-blind randomized controlled trials in the acupuncture literature, but uncontrolled series and comparison with other forms of analgesia suggest that acupuncture may be beneficial in at least 50% of patients who have failed to respond to other therapies. It is generally safe compared to other pain clinic treatments, but a number of side-effects have been reported, many of which are local to the site of needling, e.g. pneumothorax or spinal cord/root damage. As with any other invasive technique infection transmission is a potential hazard (particularly hepatitis B and HIV), but this is usually obviated by the use of disposable needles.

CHAPTER 9

ASSESSMENT OF THE PATIENT IN PAIN

INTRODUCTION

Most symptoms in medicine are assessed by means of the triad of history, examination and special investigations, which leads to a diagnosis and appropriate therapy. Pain differs from other presenting complaints in a number of ways:

- It is by definition a subjective experience
- There is often little to find on examination
- The complaint is often treated symptomatically, no 'diagnosis' having been made.

Examination and investigation form a vital part of the assessment of the patient in pain, but are principally used as objective confirmation of the patient's subjective report – the pain history.

TAKING A PAIN HISTORY

If the patient has been referred by a colleague some aspects of their history will be addressed in the referring letter, but it is preferable to obtain a 'first-hand' history from the patient (who will often see this as a reassuring sign that the pain is being taken seriously). Patients are often keen to give information on the severity of the pain, medication consumption and ideas about diagnosis (their own or those of other medical practitioners). A structured gathering of information will not miss important points. A suggested scheme is as follows:

- Age
- Site of pain – general
- Duration of complaint
- Initial precipitating event and/or relationship to significant life events
- Specific site of pain (ask patient to point)
- Radiation
- Character (may need to suggest aching, burning, shooting, stabbing, gnawing, crushing)
- Temporal pattern of pain – how many times/day/week, duration of attacks, is pain continuous? worse in morning/evening?
- Is there pain at rest?
- Is there any sleep disturbance?
- Exacerbating and relieving factors (what makes the pain better/worse?)
- Associated symptoms (always ask about neurological symptoms, numbness, weakness, paraesthesiae etc. Also ask about relevant symptoms depending on site of pain, e.g. if abdominal pain ask about GI symptoms)
- How has pain changed since onset – better/worse/same?

- Treatment so far:
  - previous medical consultations (including investigations), surgery?
  - physiotherapy
  - alternative therapies, e.g. acupuncture, chiropractic, osteopathy, herbalism, with dates and documentation of effect
- Previous and current medication (including non-prescription therapies)
  - list drugs, doses, route, timing, efficacy, side-effects, duration of therapy, reason for discontinuation
- Past medical/surgical history
- Family and social history
- Marital status (ask effect of pain on partner/sexual relationships etc.)
- Employment status patient/spouse (if out of work because of pain ask about prospects of return to work; assess motivation for this)
- If not in work, how does patient occupy self? Use this opportunity to assess how pain limits desired activity.

EXAMINATION

This should include general observation of the patient, with particular attention to:

- gait
- ability to sit comfortably in and rise from chair
- wincing/grimacing
- general mood:? anger,? confrontation
- behaviour of spouse or other attendants.

The type of further examination will depend on the site of the pain. Observation of the patient undressing may give an idea as to functional impairment. Inspection may reveal the discoloration associated with application of a hot water bottle to the affected site (erythema ab igne). Swelling (particularly of an affected joint or limb) should be noted. Comment should be made on the patient's posture. General examination must include palpation for tender areas or trigger spots. Nodules or bands may be palpable in the muscles. Painful scars should be palpated for neuromata. Neck pain or low back pain should prompt neurological examination of the upper or lower limbs respectively, noting and documenting range of movement, evidence of muscle wasting, tone, power, sensation and reflexes. Sensory testing should accompany examination of any affected part in order to determine areas of altered sensation. A number of abnormal sensory phenomena may be described by patients during examination, particularly those who have pain associated with nerve damage (Table 9.1)

TABLE 9.1 Abnormal sensory phenomena

Sensory phenomena which may be elicited on examination	
Allodynia	Pain due to a stimulus (e.g. light touch) which does not normally provoke pain
Analgesia	Absence of pain in response to stimulation which would normally be painful
Anaesthesia dolorosa	Pain in a numb area
Dysaesthesia	An unpleasant abnormal sensation, whether spontaneous or evoked
Paraesthesia	An abnormal sensation, whether spontaneous or evoked
Hyperaesthesia	Increased sensitivity to stimulation
Hyperalgesia	An increased response to a stimulus which is normally painful
Hyperpathia	Increased reaction to a stimulus and increased threshold
Hypoaesthesia	Decreased sensitivity to stimulation
Hypoalgesia	Decreased pain response to normally painful stimulus

SPECIAL TESTS AND INVESTIGATIONS

In order to quantify and qualify pain experience the clinical pain history is often supplemented by the use of pain rating scales and questionnaires. The simplest of these are the visual analogue scale (VAS), numerical rating scales (NRS), verbal rating scales (VRS) and pain drawings.

Visual analogue scale

This comprises a 10 cm line anchored by two extremes of pain: no pain on the extreme left and worst pain imaginable on the extreme right.

Patients are asked to make a mark on the line which represents their pain intensity. The score is derived by measuring the distance from the left end of the scale to the mark. Problems with this scale include difficulty of use in the elderly, conceptual difficulty for patients in understanding 'worst pain imaginable', measurement error and lack of accurate reproduction of the scale (e.g. when photocopying). A similar scale can be used to assess pain *relief*, the anchor points being *no pain relief* and *complete pain relief*.

Numerical rating scales

These involve asking the patient to rate their pain on a scale of 0 to 100 (101 possible scores). They are simple to administer, easier for the elderly to use and less prone to measurement error; 11- or 21-point scales also provide useful results.

Verbal rating scales

The most commonly used is the 4- or 5-point intensity scale. Patients are asked to indicate which word describes their pain:

- None
- Mild
- Moderate
- Severe
- Excruciating.

A numerical value (0, 1, 2, 3, 4) is then ascribed to each category for analytical purposes. However, the intervals between the categories may not be equal (e.g. greater difference between moderate and severe than between mild and moderate), making statistical analysis less valid. As with the VAS, such categorical scales can be used to assess the degree of pain relief:

- None
- Mild
- Moderate
- Complete.

A further criticism of such scales is that the small number of available categories makes them relatively insensitive.

Pain drawings

Using a human figure outline patients are asked to shade in areas corresponding to pain sensation. This provides a useful record of site and distribution of pain, and is useful in patients with more than one pain. The percentage of body surface involved in pain may be measured.

The McGill Pain Questionnare (MPQ) (Figure 9.1)

This attempts to evaluate pain qualitatively. In addition to a pain drawing and a 5-point VRS it includes a list of 78 pain adjectives divided into 20 subclasses that reflect four dimensions of pain experience, i.e. sensory, affective, evaluative (and miscellaneous). Each word is assigned a value according to its position in its subclass. Patients are asked to indicate the word(s) which best describe their pain. The MPQ can be scored by number of words chosen or their numerical value. The MPQ is available in many languages. It is time-consuming to administer and requires supervision.

A short-form MPQ (SF-MPQ) has been developed and includes 15 pain adjectives, 11 sensory and four affective, as well as a VAS and VRS. The SF-MPQ is sensitive to drug therapies.

A large number of other questionnaires are available to assess aspects of the pain experience, including disability, mood, coping, quality of life etc.

Other methods of pain assessment are summarized in Table 9.2.

McGill Pain Questionnaire

Patient's Name ______________ Date ________ Time ______ am/pm

PRI: S ______ (1–10) A ______ (11–15) E ______ (16) M ______ (17–20) PRI(T) ______ (1–20) PPI ______

1 FLICKERING QUIVERING PULSING THROBBING BEATING POUNDING	11 TIRING EXHAUSTING
2 JUMPING FLASHING SHOOTING	12 SICKENING SUFFOCATING
3 PRICKING BORING DRILLING STABBING LANCINATING	13 FEARFUL FRIGHTFUL TERRIFYING
4 SHARP CUTTING LACERATING	14 PUNISHING GRUELLING CRUEL VICIOUS KILLING
5 PINCHING PRESSING GNAWING CRAMPING CRUSHING	15 WRETCHED BLINDING
6 TUGGING PULLING WRENCHING	16 ANNOYING TROUBLESOME MISERABLE INTENSE UNBEARABLE
7 HOT BURNING SCALDING SEARING	17 SPREADING RADIATING PENETRATING PIERCING
8 TINGLING ITCHY SMARTING STINGING	18 TIGHT NUMB DRAWING SQUEEZING TEARING
9 DULL SORE HURTING ACHING HEAVY	19 COOL COLD FREEZING
10 TENDER TAUT RASPING SPLITTING	20 NAGGING NAUSEATING AGONISING DREADFUL TORTURING
	PPI 0 NO PAIN 1 MILD 2 DISCOMFORTING 3 DISTRESSING 4 HORRIBLE 5 EXCRUCIATING

BRIEF	RHYTHMIC	CONTINUOUS
MOMENTARY	PERIODIC	STEADY
TRANSIENT	INTERMITTENT	CONSTANT

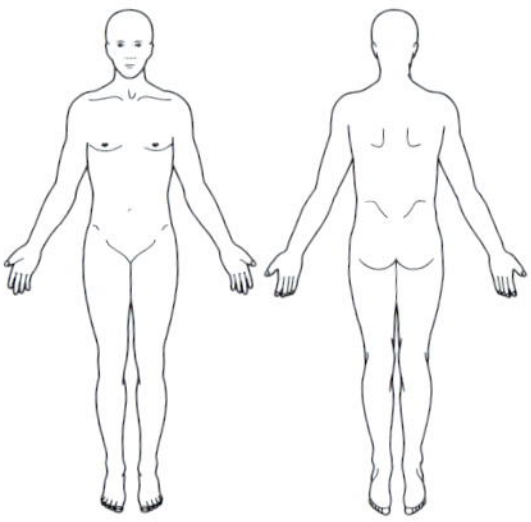

E = EXTERNAL
I = INTERNAL

COMMENTS:

Fig. 9.1 The McGill Pain Questionnaire.

TABLE 9.2 Physical methods of pain assessment

Method of assessment	*Examples*	*Comments*
Radiological	Plain X-rays, CT, MRI	Plain X-rays rarely aid diagnosis, high false positive rate, findings do not correlate with pain intensity. MRI most useful of these, especially for back pain
Diagnostic nerve blocks	Epidural block, peripheral nerve block, sympathetic nerve block	May help localize source of pain
Intravenous prognostic tests	i.v. lignocaine i.v. phentolamine	May relieve pain of neuropathic origin and suggest use of membrane stabilizing drugs May relieve pain with sympathetic component
Thermography (measures skin temperature either by means of colour change in liquid crystals or by infrared emission)		Particularly useful in Complex Regional Pain Syndrome, also for diagnosis of trigger points. Some applications in myofascial pain, nerve root pain and neuropathic pain
Measurement of autonomic variables	Pulse rate, blood pressure, skin conductance	Rarely used in chronic pain assessment
Measurement of cerebral activity	Evoked potentials, EEG	May be useful for headache
Measurement of muscle activity	EMG	Useful in some myofascial pain syndromes
Functional neuroimaging	SPECT, PET, fMRI	Research tools only

ASSESSMENT OF PAIN IN CHILDREN

Improved assessment of pain in children has greatly facilitated appropriate pain management. Accurate assessment depends on the age and developmental abilities of the child, whose experience of pain will be shaped by a number of cognitive, behavioural and emotional factors. A number of measures are now available for assessing children's pain and these can be divided into:

- physiological
- behavioural
- self-report measures.

Physiological measures

A number of quantifiable physiological variables have been used as measures of pain, including heart rate, blood pressure, respiratory rate, palmar sweating and transcutaneous oxygen. Alterations in these variables have been demonstrated during painful procedures such as heel prick and lumbar puncture. It is not known to what extent they represent a general stress response rather than the appreciation of pain. This is particularly so for measures such as increases in serum catecholamines, glucagon and corticosteroids.

Behavioural measures

Observation of the behaviour of a child in pain may aid assessment. Behaviours suggestive of discomfort, such as crying, grimacing and irritability, are assessed by a trained observer. More sophisticated quantifiable scales have been developed but are currently not in common clinical use, such as the Neonatal Facial Action Coding System where 10 facial actions are observed in response to heel prick. A limitation of behavioural scales is that it is not known to what extent certain behaviours represent response to pain rather than other forms of distress.

Self-report measures

Self-reporting is the preferred method of pain assessment in a child who can communicate verbally. Children of 18 months may be able to report the presence of pain and perhaps its location, but cannot give more information. Direct questioning is likely to yield better results than reliance on spontaneous reports.

Visual analogue scales (see above) can be used for children above the age of 5. Children who understand number concepts may also use numerical rating scales. Children may fare better with category rating scales, such as the various forms of faces scale, which consists of a series of faces (photographed or drawn) demonstrating increasing amounts of distress: the child is asked to say which face matches how they feel about their pain. Younger children may be assessed by means of concrete category scales such as the Poker Chip Tool, in which the child expresses the intensity of his pain by selecting between one and four poker chips representing 'pieces of hurt'. This latter is probably the most appropriate measure for the 4–5 year-old child.

The child's pain experience, like that of the adult, is complex, and although there have been considerable advances in pain assessment in children there is much scope for further development in the evaluation of clinical pain.

SECTION 2

ACUTE PAIN

CHAPTER 10

POSTOPERATIVE PAIN MANAGEMENT

POSTOPERATIVE PAIN, ITS MANAGEMENT AND ORGANIZATION

INTRODUCTION

The management of postoperative pain has been under scrutiny over the last decade, largely because of a failure to demonstrate improvements in pain control over the previous 30 years. Changes have been recommended and in part acted on, and the framework to provide excellent postoperative analgesia is in place.

Postoperative pain is usually due to tissue trauma and is nociceptive. As the tissue injury recovers the pain reduces. Once healing has occurred there is usually no pain. Psychological aspects have a profound impact on pain experience, and these are easily ignored.

Although it is self-limiting the pain following surgery is frequently severe, may be the most unpleasant aspect of a hospital stay, and may be the reason for remaining in hospital after surgery. Poorly treated pain contributes to postoperative complications and psychological morbidity, and may lead to future problems with persistent pain. Many studies have shown that postoperative pain is generally poorly managed. Up to 75% of patients feel moderate or severe pain in the first 24 hours after surgery; almost 90% can expect to feel a lot of pain at some point in the first 7 days postoperatively. Despite this, as little as 25% of prescribed analgesics are actually given. In various studies 100% of patients experienced some pain, and 90% had interference with sleep, meals or attention span.

CAUSES OF PAIN AFTER SURGERY

The surgical incision and tissue injury (somatic and visceral) are the commonest causes of postoperative pain. Tissue injury during surgery includes cutting, tearing, burning, stitching and traction. After surgery inflammation, ischaemia, visceral distension, traction and muscle spasm are further causes of pain.

Surgery may be associated with a variety of other pains. Minor injury may occur from lying on the operating table and from positioning of the limbs during surgery. Headache and other complaints may occur because of the ward environment. It is important that these minor pain problems are treated appropriately.

SITES AND SEVERITY

Postoperative pain is necessarily a subjective individual experience, but certain generalizations are possible:

- Major surgery is more painful than minor.
- Surface surgery is often less painful than visceral surgery.
- Tissue splitting causes less pain than tissue dividing.
- Pain on movement is worse than at rest.
- Surgery where the wound moves with respiration is more painful than peripheral surgery and is more prolonged (e.g. thoracic, upper abdominal surgery).

Many factors other than surgical site affect pain experience, including:

- Preoperative preparation and expectations
- Surgical technique (incision, use of diathermy, tissue handling, minimally invasive techniques)
- Patient positioning during surgery
- Anaesthetic technique
- Psychological aspects (fear, state and trait anxiety, neuroticism, depression, coping strategies and locus of control)
- Cultural background
- Previous experience
- Implications of pain (cancer, amputation, colostomy etc.)
- Ward environment and attitude of staff
- Diurnal variation.

These factors may also determine how individuals respond to different modes of pain relief.

WHY TREAT PAIN?

In addition to humanitarian considerations the benefits of effective pain relief include the potential to reverse the adverse physiological effects of pain and to improve the patient's psychological condition (Table 10.1). This may lead to fewer postoperative complications, earlier recovery and improved patient outcome. There is some evidence that persistent pain conditions may be modified or prevented by adequate treatment of acute pain. Good analgesia helps avoid many of these adverse sequelae

TABLE 10.1 Effects of pain

System	*Effect*	*Consequence*
General	Immobility	Lower respiratory tract infection (LRTI) Thromboembolus Muscular atrophy Pressure sores
Respiratory system	Hyperventilation Hypoventilation Fall in functional residual capacity, atelectasis collapse and consolidation Reduced diaphragmatic activity Inability to tolerate physiotherapy	LRTI Tissue acidosis Hypoxaemia
Cardiovascular system	Hypertension Tachycardia Vasoconstriction	Increased cardiac work Decreased oxygen delivery Ischaemia and infarction
Neuroendocrine system	Increased stress response (increased catecholamines and catabolism) Immunosuppression Peripheral and central nervous sensitization	Increased circulating fats Decreased gut mobility Decreased healing Increased infection risk Risk of persistent pain
Gastrointestinal system	Nausea Ileus	Prolonged intravenous support Dehydration Electrolyte imbalances Malnutrition
Psychological	Anxiety Fear Disappointment Anger Depression	Loss of confidence (in self and in carers) Loss of therapeutic relationship

METHODS OF PAIN RELIEF

These are summarized in Table 10.2.

APPROPRIATE ANALGESIA

Complete analgesia may be achieved in all postoperative patients by the use of high-dose opioids and regional analgesia. However, this is unnecessary and inappropriate. Much postoperative pain can be easily controlled by short periods of opioid analgesia or other agents. Simplicity is preferable, and complex techniques should only be used if beneficial.

TABLE 10.2 Commonly used methods of postoperative pain relief

Methods of pain relief	*Examples*
Physical	Elevation of injured part Transcutaneous nerve stimulation (TENS) Acupuncture Cooling
Drug treatment	Opioids Non-steroidal anti-inflammatory drugs (NSAIDs) Paracetamol Inhalation agents
Local anaesthetic techniques	Topical Infiltration Nerve blocks Regional or plexus blocks
Psychological	Information and explanation Reassurance Emotional support Behavioural methods

MODERN APPROACHES

The neurophysiological sequelae of pain are discussed in Chapter 1. An understanding of the physiology of pain has given rise to the concepts of pre-emptive analgesia and balanced analgesia.

PRE-EMPTIVE ANALGESIA

Hypersensitivity has been demonstrated both peripherally and centrally in several species, including humans. Laboratory work suggests that analgesia prior to injury reduces or abolishes hypersensitivity. For example, small doses of opioid before noxious stimulus reduces hyperexcitability. In vitro it can be abolished. Once hypersensitivity is established large doses are needed to have any effect. Similar results are demonstrated using afferent blockade with local anaesthesia. NSAIDs may also have similar effect. This is the basis of pre-emptive analgesia.

Clinical studies in humans have been disappointing. Reasons for this include poor study design and the fact that postsurgical pain is different from brief experimental pain used in laboratory investigations.

Many questions remain unanswered: it is unclear whether preventing peripheral, central or both forms of hypersensitivity is the most important strategy. The relative importance of the nociceptive barrage from surgery and from ongoing postoperative pain remains unclear. Whether sensitization is the same for visceral and somatic injury is not known. In addition, the role of inhibitory pain mechanisms is often neglected. Noxious stimuli and tissue injury activate a number of physiological changes that oppose the hypersensitivity process and may act to modulate pain transmission. These include:

- expression of peripheral and dorsal horn opioid receptors
- increased descending modulation
- unregulation of GABA and glycine (inhibitory) systems
- reduction during inflammation, cholecystokinin, which acts as a brake on opioid analgesia.

It is not known to what extent pre-emptive analgesia prevents the operation of these inhibitory mechanisms.

Effective pre-emptive analgesia should produce lower pain scores, a longer interval to the first request for analgesia and a reduction in total analgesic consumption. Clinical sequalae of pain might also reduce. Although this area continues to stimulate much research, the clinical benefits are yet to be realized.

BALANCED ANALGESIA

Ideal analgesia often cannot be achieved with any single agent: this goal is more frequently achieved with multimodal analgesia. Instead of relying on one class of drug to treat pain, a variety of drug groups, acting at different points in the pain path, are used. Smaller doses of each drug are used and dose-dependent side effects are reduced while analgesia is improved.

For mild – moderate pain a combination of NSAID and opioid is frequently used, in addition to peroperative local infiltration or nerve block.

For major surgery and severe pain local anaesthetic techniques (such as a continuous epidural infusion) combined with an opioid given systemically or into the regional infusion are appropriate. NSAIDs may also be added.

Undoubtedly balanced analgesia can provide near-perfect pain relief, but it is demanding of resources and nursing time, and local guide lines may require monitoring in high-dependency units.

ORGANIZATIONAL ASPECTS OF POSTOPERATIVE ANALGESIA

WHY DOES POSTOPERATIVE PAIN MANAGEMENT FAIL?

- Patient expectations are generally low. Patients do not expect analgesia to fully relieve pain: most believe that it should allow them to lie comfortably in bed. Many patients delay requesting analgesia until pain is severe. Some believe pain is necessary for recovery and should not be mentioned. Because of poor expectations satisfaction scores may be high in the face of high levels of pain.

- Staff expectations and ignorance also often inhibit good pain management. Nurses fear addiction in patients on opioid medication. Less than half of doctors and nurses believe that analgesia should relieve pain completely. Junior doctors are often poorly educated about analgesia, and more aware of the side-effects of analgesics than their efficacy. Other misconceptions include the belief that postoperative pain is inevitable, that patients object to an injection more than to continuing pain, and that patients cannot be in pain without objective signs. **NB: when more than one dose is prescribed the lower dose is given more frequently than the larger**.
- Organization and resource allocation for pain management has traditionally had low priority on postoperative wards. Pain assessments are often not recorded and the allocation of time to administer analgesia often restricted to nurses' 'drug rounds'. Administering opioid analgesia entails a delay while drugs are obtained from secure cupboards and checked by two qualified staff.
- Pharmacokinetics and pharmacodynamic aspects. The traditional intramuscular opioid PRN prescription allows a fixed dose (often too little) of one drug to be delivered at a fixed interval (often too long). If analgesia is inadequate or short-lived, prolonged pain results. Blood levels of drug fluctuate and may either reach toxic levels or never reach an analgesic level. Intramuscular injections rely on absorption of the drug into the bloodstream, and this is dependent on muscle blood flow. In hypovolaemia and hypothermia, both of which are frequent after surgery, blood flow may be reduced and absorption delayed. Absorption also varies with the site of injection and, in the case of pethidine, repeated use of the same site reduces bioavailability.

Interindividual variations are also found in:

- minimum effective analgesic concentration (MEAC)
- drug concentrations that produce side-effects
- rates of metabolism
- relative proportion of morphine metabolized to the important analgesically active metabolite morphine-6-glucuronide (M6G).

Because of these many variations it is not surprising that studies to determine which patient characteristics predict analgesic requirements in adults have shown no correlation with patient weight, height or body surface area. There is an inverse correlation with age, analgesic requirements reducing by approximately 50% between the ages of 30 and 70. Differences between the requirements of men and women are so small as to be ignored.

A fixed attitude to analgesic requirements will lead to failure in many patients because of pharmacokinetic variability.

PRINCIPLES FOR IMPROVEMENT OF ANALGESIA

- Education of patient, nursing and medical staff in pain management and analgesic techniques
- Individualized analgesia: patient-centred pain prescriptions to reflect the markedly variable response of individuals to the same surgical procedure
- Organizational restructuring so that the provision of analgesia is part of the scheduled work pattern (the named nurse policy and regular pain assessment are included in this, but adequate staffing levels are essential)
- Preventative analgesia to prevent or control pain before it becomes a problem
- Multimodal analgesia to improve efficacy without increasing side-effects
- Regular assessment of pain and side-effects, so that pain is detected, treatment can be rationalized and the effect of treatment observed
- Patient participation or administration where possible
- Attention to psychological aspects.

THE ACUTE PAIN SERVICE

An acute pain service (APS) has been introduced in many hospitals in recent years. Its role is to improve the provision of analgesia for patients suffering from acute pain, usually postoperatively. It is uncommon for the APS to be able to review all postoperative patients, but the service should be available to anyone who needs it. Patients using opioid infusions and epidurals are commonly seen.

In some hospitals the APS also oversees analgesia for non-surgical acute pain, such as sickle cell crises and acute back and abdominal pain.

Useful members of the APS may include anaesthetists, a trained nurse specialist, a pharmacist and a psychologist.

Roles

- Supervision or surveillance of postoperative pain and analgesia: safety and efficacy
- Education of patients, nursing and medical staff in pain management. The use of protocols allows the delegation of much routine pain management to ward staff and maintains a consistent approach.
- Audit of pain management.

Referral

Patients who might benefit from referral to the APS should have analgesic expectations and techniques discussed preoperatively. The provision of good analgesia in the recovery room is important as it allows a chosen technique to be tested and established, its immediate safety to be assessed, and it might be hoped to raise patients' expectations by demonstrating good analgesia.

Organization

The organization of the APS should provide 24-hour support to the wards but **should not exclude other staff working with the patient**.

EFFECT OF THE INTRODUCTION OF AN APS

The introduction of an APS produces several benefits:

- More generous use of analgesics
- Improved analgesia (particularly reduced frequency of severe pain)
- Reduced frequency of the side-effects of analgesia (e.g. nausea and vomiting, sedation, hypotension)
- Reduced frequency of the sequelae of poor analgesia
- Increased staff knowledge and altered attitudes
- Safe introduction of novel analgesic techniques
- Improved patient satisfaction
- Improved staff satisfaction with analgesia.

In late 1994 43% of hospitals reported having an APS. This was estimated to be a tenfold increase over the previous 5 years.

ASSESSMENT OF PAIN

In order to treat pain effectively it is necessary to assess it (see Chapter 9). Because of its subjective nature, **pain is most effectively assessed by means of self-report**.

The measure must be reproducible. For postoperative pain complicated scoring systems identifying the type of pain and affective and emotional components are rarely needed. More important is to assess the severity of the pain, regularly.

Visual analogue scales have been used, but verbal ratings are probably more readily understood by the majority of patients. A cycle of assessment, response and reassessment is central to the effective treatment of pain (and the prevention of side-effects). There is no benefit in documenting the extent of suffering if no effective action is then taken. It is useful to chart pain scores graphically to identify progress. This also facilitates audit and research.

Side-effects (e.g. nausea) should be recorded so that the balance of analgesia and side-effects can be established.

Analgesia that produces mild pain at rest with severe pain during activity does not allow the maximum rate of recovery after major surgery. Pain should be assessed:

in the first 24 hours

- during coughing and physiotherapy
- during leg movement;

after 24 hours

- during coughing and physiotherapy
- during mobilization.

Analgesia should not be considered satisfactory unless it is effective during these activities.

SAFETY MONITORING

As well as assessing the efficacy of analgesia, monitoring should detect side-effects that may be unpleasant for the patient or potentially dangerous. The type of monitoring depends on the likelihood of adverse effects occurring. For all patients assessment should initially be very frequent while analgesia is established in the early postoperative period. If no problems are found monitoring may be progressively reduced to a minimum. Whenever a problem does occur increased vigilance and intensity of monitoring are required.

Vital signs should be regularly monitored in all patients following surgery, irrespective of their analgesic management. Although this is principally to detect postsurgical complications the vital signs may alert to the possibility of inadequate analgesia or developing complications.

As opioids are the mainstay of postoperative pain management the side-effects associated with their use must be sought, particularly the following:

- *Nausea and vomiting*. As this side-effect is so common (occurring in up to 40% of patients after surgery) efforts should be made to prevent it, particularly as rescue medication may be ineffective. When nausea and vomiting preclude effective analgesia consideration should be given to changing to another type of analgesia.
- *Sedation and airway obstruction* are common after surgery owing to a combination of recovery from anaesthetic agents and the effects of opioids and other sedative medications. Sedative medications interact with each

other. Mild sedation may be pleasant for the patient and is not harmful. Increasing sedation or a patient who is unrousable by simple means may indicate developing complications (e.g. syphoning from an opioid infusion, migration of an epidural catheter) and causes its own adverse effects (immobility, poor respiratory effort, lack of cooperation and reduced airway protection). Airway obstruction produces hypoxia more quickly than respiratory depression, and arousal is an important factor in maintaining pharyngeal muscle tone and hence airway patency. When opioids are combined with benzodiazepines, the likelihood of airway obstruction increases. Obese patients are especially at risk following major surgery. N.B. opioid induced respiratory depression is commonly preceded by increasing sedation.

- *Respiratory depression*. This is most frequently assessed by counting respiratory rate (neither sensitive nor specific), so should be supplemented by observation of chest movements and, where possible, continuous pulse oximetry, particularly for high-risk patients (obesity, abdominal surgery, lung disease, ischaemic cardiac disease). **Apnoea monitors** are necessary for neonates receiving opioid infusions.

Monitoring the device

Equipment malfunction is a less common cause of adverse event than user error.

Where devices such as infusion pumps are used safety checks should be made as follows:

- Correct drug?
- Correct administration rate?
- Device appropriately powered?
- Device safely positioned?
- Syringe mounted correctly?
- Evidence of tampering?
- Appropriate quantity of drug delivered since previous check?
- Check infusion site.

ANALGESIC TECHNIQUES AND AGENTS

INTRODUCTION

Much of the information in this section is discussed in Chapters 2–7. Particular problems associated with the use of various techniques in the postoperative period are discussed here. The techniques of patient-controlled (PCA) and spinal (particularly epidural) analgesia are discussed separately. Supervision of and education about these techniques forms the bulk of acute pain service activity in many hospitals. **It is important to remember that when these techniques are not available there is much that can be done by sensible use of common analgesic agents**.

OPIOIDS

Potent opioids

Opioids are the mainstay of postoperative pain management. The advantages of opioid analgesia are:

- It is widely available
- It is effective by many routes
- There are few if any absolute contraindications.

Disadvantages are:

- Frequent minor side-effects
- Occasional severe or life-threatening side-effects
- Considerable variations in patient response
- Controlled drugs, so delay in administration.

The route of administration has relevance postoperatively.

ORAL TABLETS AND SOLUTIONS

Absorption is dependent on the drug reaching the small bowel. Postoperative ileus is common and opioids themselves contribute to gastric stasis and vomiting. As a result drug delivery is unpredictable. A large quantity of oral opioid may accumulate in the stomach during this period of stasis. When gut motility resumes an effective overdose may be absorbed by the small bowel.

For these reasons potent oral opioids are generally unsuitable for treating early postoperative pain. During the later stages of hospital stay oral opioids may be useful.

RECTAL

This route can be used when patients are nauseated or the oral route is not established. Rectal medication is unpleasant for both nurses and patients, and may not be favoured by surgeons after gastrointestinal surgery.

INTRAMUSCULAR

This is the conventional route for postoperative opioid administration. The pharmacokinetics are discussed elsewhere, but **in the cold, hypovolaemic patient poor muscle perfusion leads to unpredictable absorption**.

INTRAVENOUS

Bolus

The intravenous route is the simplest by which to establish rapid and effective analgesia (e.g. in the recovery ward or casualty department), which may then be maintained by another method or by further titrated boluses when pain returns. With suitable training and observation the technique is suitable for use in general wards and by nursing staff.

Infusion

Steady-state drug concentrations allow a constant level of analgesia and may be used to prevent rather than treat pain. However, analgesic requirements are not constant and notably reduce as time progresses. As a result constant-rate infusions are associated with a high incidence of clinically important respiratory depression. Although infusion devices are cheaper than PCA devices and are easy to use, skilled nurse supervision and several infusion adjustments may be needed to maintain effective, safe analgesia.

Patient-controlled analgesia is discussed below.

Peripheral administration of opioids

A relatively recent discovery was the demonstration of opioid receptors (μ and δ) on primary afferent neurones both at nerve terminals and along the axon. This appears to occur particularly in inflamed tissues, and occurs rapidly after the onset of inflammation. The opioid receptors may block the transmission of nociceptive information by altering transduction and blocking action potential propagation. In animal studies opioids applied to the site of inflammation are effective. This development raises the possibility of using opioids that are active in the periphery only. This might reduce centrally mediated side-effects such as respiratory depression.

Several studies have examined the efficacy of peripheral opioid analgesia in humans with disappointing results, except for intra-articular morphine administration where effective, long lasting analgesia is reported.

WEAK OPIOIDS AND COMPOUND ANALGESIC PREPARATIONS

Weak opioids include codeine, dihydrocodeine and dextropropoxyphene. In oral preparations weak opioids are frequently combined with paracetamol. When the two are combined pain relief is slightly better than with paracetamol alone, but side-effects are increased. These combination preparations are frequently prescribed for moderate pain such as after day-case surgery or on discharge from hospital. The dose of paracetamol in preparations varies and those that allow a dose of 1 g paracetamol up to four times a day are more effective than those with lower doses. As the duration of action of paracetamol and of these opioids is not the same, it is logical to avoid combination analgesics and prescribe them separately. This should be balanced against the likely reduction in compliance. Efficacy for moderate pain may be less than with NSAIDs and is certainly improved if an NSAID is added.

NON-STEROIDAL ANTI-INFLAMMATORY DRUGS (NSAIDs)

NSAIDs are particularly effective for soft-tissue damage and pain from bone injury where an anti-inflammatory effect may be important (e.g. orthopaedic and dental pain). They are effective analgesics for minor and some moderate pain, and useful adjuncts in severe pain in conjunction with other techniques such as PCA or local anaesthetic block. The combination of paracetamol and a NSAID is more effective than either alone.

A wide variety of NSAIDs are now available by a variety of routes. The incidence of side-effects correlates well with each drug's ability to inhibit the enzyme cyclooxygenase 1.

Routes of administration:

- Oral
- Rectal
- Buccal
- Intramuscular
- Intravenous
- Topical
- Intra-articular.

The advantages of NSAIDs for postoperative pain are:

- Effective analgesia in mild to moderate pain
- Opioid-sparing effect in severe pain
- Minimal effect on vital signs
- No risk of sedation or respiratory depression
- Long duration of action

- Available by several routes
- Not restricted by Controlled Drug regulations.

Disadvantages:

- Side-effects may make them unsuitable for a proportion of patients
- Inadequate analgesia in severe pain
- Delay in onset of analgesia, even when given intravenously
- Potential risk of perioperative bleeding
- Potential for peptic ulceration
- Potential for impaired renal blood flow in hypovolaemia
- Considered by some to contraindicate regional blockade.

PARACETAMOL

Like NSAIDs, paracetamol affects prostaglandin synthesis, particularly in the brain. It does not block cyclo-oxygenase-1 or -2. It may inhibit a different subtype of the enzyme in the central nervous system (COX3). It has analgesic and antipyretic but no anti-inflammatory effects. It is effective alone in mild pain and is a useful adjunct in moderate or severe pain. Maximal benefit is gained when it is given regularly to its maximum safe dose of 4 g/day. In conventional doses side-effects are extremely rare. It is available as oral or rectal preparations.

LESS FREQUENTLY USED ANALGESICS

TRAMADOL

Tramadol, a synthetic analogue of codeine, has both opioid and non-opioid analgesic actions. It can be given orally by intramuscular and intravenous injection.

Reports of efficacy equal to that of morphine are balanced by reports of very poor efficacy. It should be regarded as an analgesic for moderate pain. It is not currently a controlled drug but the CSM recommends its use only for short duration, for moderate or severe pain, and with great caution in those with a history of drug or alcohol dependence. Nausea and vomiting are common.

MEPTAZINOL

This rarely used centrally acting synthetic drug has opioid and non-opioid actions and is associated with central cholinergic effects. Its action is antagonized by naloxone and anticholinergic agents. It is claimed to be associated with a lower incidence of respiratory depression than morphine, but nausea and vomiting are common. It has a length of action of between 2 and 7 hours.

NEFOPAM

This is a non-opioid analgesic with intermediate potency. As with many analgesics some studies have found it as effective as potent opioids for moderate pain. Others have found it ineffective. Although a significant proportion of patients will not tolerate the drug it remains an alternative for those who are unable to take opioids or NSAIDs. The dose is 60 mg orally or 20 mg intramuscularly up to three times a day. Side-effects include antimuscarinic and sympathomimetic symptoms.

STEROIDS

Steroids may reduce pain through an anti-inflammatory effect and may also have specific analgesic effects. Dexamethasone reduces swelling and pain after dental surgery. Intra-articular steroids are reported to provide effective and prolonged analgesia after arthroscopy.

LOCAL ANAESTHETIC TECHNIQUES

Local anaesthetic techniques have a number of advantages when used for postoperative pain management:

- Excellent analgesia may be achieved at rest and on movement
- Infiltration and superficial nerve blocks are simple and rapidly effective
- Techniques may be used for all age groups with few contraindications
- Minimal systemic side-effects if recommended dosage observed
- Avoidance of the side-effects of opioids (particularly preservation of respiratory function) and NSAIDs
- Muscle spasm reduced
- Duration can be prolonged by the use of catheters.

Disadvantages:

- Infiltration or nerve location may be uncomfortable for the patient
- Limited duration of effect of currently used local anaesthetics as single injections
- Sensory blockade may allow further trauma if site not protected. Secondary injury must be avoided
- Motor blockade may be unpleasant or even immobilizing
- Intense analgesia may mask clinical signs of other painful complications (e.g. compartment syndrome, angina)
- Unwanted sympathetic blockade (hypotension with spinal techniques)
- Risk of systemic toxicity from absolute overdose or misplaced local anaesthetic (intravascular, intrathecal)
- Risk of temporary or permanent neurological damage (rare)

- Specific complications may prevent bilateral blocks being performed (e.g. intercostal, or supraclavicular blocks and pneumothorax).

Many of these disadvantages may be avoided by good technique.

GENERAL CONSIDERATIONS AND CONTRAINDICATIONS

The use of local anaesthetic techniques has risen in the last decade, particularly for day-case and paediatric surgery. In all cases the nature of the performance of the block, side-effects and complications should be discussed with the patient before surgery. Patient refusal or lack of understanding is the strongest contraindication. Sepsis at the site of intended injection is also a contraindication. Pre-existing neurological deficits must be balanced against the proposed benefit of the technique and should be meticulously documented. Coagulation abnormalities reduce the margin of safety and are a contraindication for some blocks. As overdose or inadvertent intravascular injection causes cardiovascular collapse and convulsions, expertise and resuscitation equipment must be immediately available.

TYPES OF LOCAL ANAESTHESIA

Topical

EMLA (eutectic mixture of local anaesthetics) cream combines lignocaine 2.5% and prilocaine 2.5% and is effective topically but may cause vasoconstriction. Useful analgesia may require 30 minutes' application. Amethocaine gel (4%) has faster onset, a more prolonged effect, and causes vasodilatation. Local hypersensitivity may occur. Both are used primarily for venepuncture and are applied under occlusive dressings. They may be used on burns or sites of split-skin grafting.

Topical bupivacaine may be used peroperatively on split-skin graft donor sites.

Topical amethocaine may provide effective analgesia following squint surgery and other forms of eye surgery.

Infiltration

Wounds may be infiltrated at the end of surgery but it is unclear which layers of tissue are most effectively infiltrated. Infiltration techniques are effective for many small wounds and for intermediate wounds, such as after hernia repairs. Efficacy has been harder to demonstrate for larger incisions covering more dermatomes, such as major abdominal and thoracic wounds. Local infiltration does not block deeper structures and visceral innervation, which may account for its small effect after major surgery. There is little evidence to support a pre-emptive effect of infiltration before incision. Wound healing should not be affected by local anaesthetics as most are vasodilators, and wound infection should not result as local anaesthetics have some antibacterial activity. Care should, however, be taken, with contaminated wounds, where the volume of local anaesthesia may disrupt wound apposition (e.g. round the ankle), and in the use of vasoconstrictors. Many surgeons remain resistant to the technique.

The effect of infiltration is short-lived but may be increased by insertion of a catheter into or near the wound. The block may then be prolonged with infusion or even patient controlled administration.

NB: Spraying the wound with local anaesthetic is generally ineffective.

Nerve blockade

For large wounds toxic doses of local anaesthetic may be required to provide analgesia by infiltration. Superficial nerves may be blocked at a site distant to the wound, which reduces the dose needed and avoids infiltration of the surgical site.

Suitable nerves for blockade are listed in Table 10.3. The techniques are particularly suitable for children.

TABLE 10.3 Nerve blocks for postoperative pain

Nerve block	*Type of surgery*
Commonly performed	
Ilioinguinal, iliohypogastric and genitofemoral	Inguinal and femoral hernia
Dorsal nerve of the penis	Penis
Femoral	Front of thigh above patella
Lateral cutaneous nerve of the thigh	Lateral thigh
Ankle block (5 nerves)	Foot
Digital (ring block)	Digit
Intercostal	Chest or abdominal wall
Less common	
Greater auricular	Pinna
Supraorbital and supratrochlear	Forehead
Infraorbital	Lower eyelid and upper lip
Inferior alveolar nerve	Lower teeth
Mental nerve	Lower lip
Ulnar (at elbow or wrist)	Ulnar aspect of hand
Radial (at elbow or wrist)	Radial side of back of hand
Median (at elbow or wrist)	Palm of radial 3 fingers

Other nerves may be blocked for postsurgical analgesia but are less accessible and therefore infrequently used. These include sciatic and pudendal nerves.

Plexus blockade

Groups of nerves emerging from the spinal foramina form plexuses that may be blocked within their fascial compartments. These produce analgesia over a wide region of dermatomes (Table 10.4). Significant sympathetic and motor blockade is usual. The techniques require more expertise than superficial nerve blocks, and may be made more effective and safer by the skilled use of a nerve stimulator. Knowledge of anatomy, careful technique and gentle treatment of tissues should minimize the risk of nerve damage. Plexus blocks are particularly suitable for prolongation by inserting a catheter for repeat bolus or continuous infusion.

TABLE 10.4 Plexus blocks for postoperative pain

Plexus blockade	*Region of analgesia*
Superficial cervical	Anterior neck (including carotid and thyroid surgery)
Interscalene approach to brachial plexus	Upper arm and shoulder
Supraclavicular approach to brachial plexus	Elbow and arm
Axillary approach to brachial plexus	Lower arm and hand
Femoral 3 in 1 or iliacus block of lumbar plexus	Femoral surgery and lateral thigh

OTHER BLOCKS

Other regional techniques which may be useful postoperatively include paravertebral and interpleural blocks.

Paravertebral block involves the injection or insertion of a catheter into the paravertebral space. It is particularly indicated following thoracotomy, its main advantage being that it blocks the posterior primary ramus (innervating the paravertebral skin and costovertebral joints), which intercostal blockade misses. As it does not cause bilateral sympathetic blockade the risk of hypotension is less than with epidural techniques. It is suitable for analgesia after any form of unilateral thoracic or abdominal surgery. Bilateral blockade may be performed but there is risk of pneumothorax, and as bilateral sympathetic blockade occurs any advantage over epidural analgesia is lost. Side-effects include pneumothorax, venous puncture, epidural spread, hypotension and systemic toxicity.

Interpleural analgesia is produced by insertion of local anaesthetic into the pleural cavity. This may be performed percutaneously or at thoracotomy, and a catheter is usually inserted. The pleural space is bathed in local anaesthetic, providing widespread intercostal blockade. It may be used for thoracotomy, cholecystectomy or nephrectomy. Results are very variable and it is a technique used only by a few. With the percutaneous technique there is a significant risk of pneumothorax.

Intra-articular injection of local anaesthetic after arthroscopy (particularly of the knee) is widely practised. A variety of doses, volumes and additives have been used. Results of studies are conflicting.

Epidural analgesia is discussed below.

INHALATIONAL AGENTS

ENTONOX

Entonox (nitrous oxide 50%, oxygen 50%) is the only agent available on wards for inhalational analgesia. Because of low blood solubility it produces rapid onset of analgesia without loss of consciousness. Analgesia starts within 60 seconds of use and is maximal at 120 seconds. Offset is equally fast. It is useful for brief painful procedures (e.g. burns dressing, removal of drains). It should not be used for prolonged periods as this may lead to bone marrow depression. Use in patients with pneumothorax or pneumoperitoneum leads to complications through expansion of the gas. Scavenging is necessary, as there are concerns over its effect on fertility, fetal development and environmental safety. Entonox is used extensively in labour and is discussed further in Chapter 13.

PSYCHOLOGICAL APPROACHES

Although most acute pain is nociceptive (physiological) the integration and response to it will have affective, cognitive and social components. Attention to these aspects can lead to a considerable reduction in pain and suffering. Psychological intervention may alter not only what the patient feels but also the response to those sensations. The approach requires skill to be practised effectively, although some aspects (explanation, comfort, open discussion) will be incorporated by the caring approach of the 'good doctor' and 'good nurse'. The particular psychological make-up of the individual will determine what coping strategies he or she adopts, whether adjunctive psychological approaches are useful, and may affect which forms of pain relief are effective (see section on Patient-controlled analgesia).

Staff training in these aspects of patient preparation and support would improve the care most patients receive during their hospital stay. There are significant resource implications for both the training and the time taken to practise these techniques.

Interventions may be classified as follows:

- *Explanation* of what will be done and what will be felt. Explanation increases knowledge, which may reduce fear. Strategies to cope (with pain) may be planned in the light of this information. The patient becomes less passive and is able to achieve some control and anticipate and participate in events. Written information, audio tapes and videos may be useful methods of providing information. A tour of an intensive care or postoperative ward is useful.
- Methods to *alter pain behaviour*. (Learned and structured reactions to pain) include tools to increase mental relaxation, calmness and muscle relaxation. The ability to perform these learned behaviours in spite of pain may reduce patients' distress.
- *Cognitive* approaches relate to attitude and thought processes. A patient may concentrate on positive rather than negative thoughts, and attempt rational rather than irrational responses. Morale is improved and passivity lessened.
- *Psychotherapy* explores feelings and beliefs. Anxieties and emotions are discussed in an attempt to increase the person's understanding of how they think and respond. A greater understanding of self may develop.

Explanation, behavioural and cognitive approaches have been shown by controlled trials to reduce postoperative pain, and analgesic use is reduced by each of these forms of psychological intervention. Reduced distress, improved satisfaction, reduced stay and better measures of wellbeing have also been shown.

HYPNOSIS

This is another approach that may be very effective in self-selected groups, but requires time and training. Not all patients are amenable to this form of therapy.

PHYSICAL METHODS OF PAIN RELIEF

Transcutaneous nerve stimulation

Although several studies have concluded that TENS is an effective adjunct for postoperative pain relief few of these were randomized controlled trials and definitive evidence of efficacy is lacking. Systematic review of well conducted controlled trials found no evidence that TENS is effective for postoperative analgesia. A major advantage is that there are no known adverse effects.

Acupuncture

Acupuncture is frequently used outside the UK, and some studies report impressive results. It requires skill, time and acceptance by the patient. Electro-acupuncture and moxibustion are variants.

Localized wound cooling with surface cooling devices has also been shown to be effective in producing analgesia, but controlled studies have not been performed. It is not likely to have much effect on visceral pain and may impede wound healing.

Cryoanalgesia

In this technique a cooling device (cryoprobe) is applied under direct vision during surgery to a sensory nerve, most often an intercostal nerve at thoracotomy. Application to mixed or motor nerves must be avoided as this would lead to prolonged paralysis of supplied muscles. Temperatures of –70°C are achieved and axonal function is disrupted. Analgesia is produced by deafferentation, but even with good denervation analgesia may not be complete. Nerve regeneration takes place over a number of months and may lead to persistent pain. Prolonged anaesthesia in the distribution of the nerve may be unpleasant.

PATIENT-CONTROLLED ANALGESIA (PCA)

This term refers to the administration of analgesia by the patient. A variety of routes and drug groups have been used. The intravenous administration of opioids is the most common technique.

Patient-controlled intravenous analgesia has been used for over 30 years. A mechanical or electrical device allows the patient to self-administer small boluses of intravenous analgesia. The **bolus** size is conventionally fixed and a **lock-out period** is built into the system during which the device is refractory to further patient demands. A **background infusion** may be added, and limitations on consumption may be programmed into some machines.

The basis for the technique is that a feedback loop is produced which allows the patient to titrate analgesia to their own MEAC (minimum effective anaesthetic concentration). Delays in delivery are eliminated and small frequent doses of rapid onset reduce the fluctuations in plasma concentration seen with intramuscular analgesia. Excessive demands lead to sedation, which precludes further patient-initiated demands, so creating a safe system.

CHOICE OF DRUG

Morphine is the most widely used drug for PCA. Onset of effect is within 5 minutes, allowing the patient to rapidly appreciate the effect of a bolus. The optimum demand dose and lockout period vary for each drug, but are not established for all drugs. Therefore the efficacy of other drugs compared to morphine is inconsistently reported and difficult to interpret, as ideal regimens may not be used. Diamorphine produces similar efficacy; in some reports pethidine is less effective and less well tolerated. Good analgesia can be obtained with fentanyl.

DOSE

Bolus size must be set so that the patient appreciates an effect after each bolus, with minimum adverse symptoms. Reported doses of morphine range from 0.1 to 4 mg. Several studies have demonstrated that 1 mg boluses of morphine produce the fewest failures and the fewest requirements to alter the bolus size. The same bolus size will not suit all patients, however: inadequate analgesia with frequent demands may require an increase in bolus size; excessive sedation despite infrequent boluses should trigger a reduction in bolus size. Increases of 50–100% or decreases of 50% are appropriate.

LOCKOUT PERIOD

This should be timed to allow the patient to appreciate the maximal effect of the last bolus before a further demand is made. It should also allow analgesia to be regained after periods of sleep or interruption. Reported lockout durations for morphine range from 1 to 10 minutes. Despite theoretical dangers there is no clear evidence that a lockout duration as low as 1 minute is more dangerous than one of 5 minutes. The self-imposed lockout period chosen by many patients is often well in excess of that chosen by the prescriber. In spite of poor analgesia these patients will not increase their demand frequency.

INFUSION

Imposing a fixed rate of drug delivery (an infusion) to a patient is counter to the premises of PCA and removes safety from the feedback loop: excessive sedation will not terminate a fixed infusion. Many studies have examined the place of background infusions during PCA: a few have demonstrated improved analgesia but most have not, and the technique is associated with a greater incidence of side-effects. Background infusion is not recommended.

EQUIPMENT

A wide variety of devices is available. These vary from simple disposable mechanical devices to complex electronic programmable, reusable machines. Each has several components in common.

- Storage of the drug is in a reservoir in the form of a disposable syringe or bag of 50–250 ml.
- Driving system. The reservoir is driven by an electronic or mechanical system. Motorized pumps include plunger depressors for syringes and rotor or peristaltic systems for devices with reservoir bags. Mechanical devices may rely on finger pressure to empty a small reservoir containing

the drug bolus. This refills from the main drug reservoir by using stored mechanical energy from an elastomeric balloon or spring-loaded syringe.
- Power. Electronic devices require mains or battery power; most mechanical devices do not.
- Programming may be complex in electronic devices, with variations in bolus size, rate of administration, lockout period, background infusion and dose limits. There may be clinician override. In mechanical devices there is routinely no variability in programming and system characteristics are intrinsic to the device.
- Displays and data collection vary from none to sophisticated displays of drug regimens and usage. Hourly demands and drug delivery may be recorded. Information may be downloaded via a computer interface.
- The patient interface is usually a handheld button (handset). A single press activates the machine electronically or pneumatically. Early devices incorporated a safety requirement for two presses within one second to initiate a demand, but this is now rare. In some mechanical devices pressure directly on the delivery reservoir releases the bolus. Adaptation can usually be achieved for those who find buttons difficult to depress, such as patients with arthritis, children and the physically disabled.
- Safety features include programmable aspects. However, the reservoir containing large doses of controlled drug should be tamperproof and the programming should be protected by code or key.
- Alarms may be incorporated to identify occlusion, a nearly empty reservoir, tampering, malfunction or power failure. The device may be linked to a respiratory monitor that activates an alarm and simultaneously disables the device if respiratory depression is detected.

SAFETY

Most machines have safety devices built in. Although these may fail, **most serious incidents associated with PCA are due to human error**. Incorrect programming and preparation of syringes is common. Lack of familiarity with the technique and equipment make this more likely: PCA devices should therefore only be set up or altered by those appropriately trained. A standardized hospital protocol, prepacked sterile syringes and standardized monitoring policies should further increase safety.

All PCA delivery systems should be designed to prevent the possibility of syphonage or reflux of solution. This may be achieved by using a dedicated site of intravenous access or a one-way valve incorporating an anti-syphon device. PCA devices should be mounted horizontally and above the level of the patient's heart.

Regimens without a background infusion increase safety but do not assure it. Programmable safety limits, such as a 4-hour drug limit, have not been shown to improve safety and are of little benefit.

PSYCHOLOGICAL ASPECTS

The essential premise of PCA is that control of analgesia is given to the patient. It has been assumed that when patients are given control they will titrate medication until they achieve a pain-free state; they do not always do so (see below).

It is a prerequisite of PCA that the patient understands the principles of the technique (at its simplest, that pressing a button when in pain will relieve that pain). The technique is not successful for all patients.

PATIENT'S PERCEPTIONS OF PCA

- The ability to take control of analgesia is not reported by all patients to be a benefit.
- Fears of overdose and a self-imposed maximum demand rate have been noted.
- The end-point of titration is not necessarily pain relief: patients may press the button for a variety of reasons, including because they were told to, and to demonstrate the equipment to visitors.
- Reasons for not pressing the button include the association with side-effects, a belief that pain is necessary, and fear of overdose or addiction.

CLINICAL EFFICACY

There is no doubt that PCA is popular with patients and very high levels of satisfaction are reported when it is used. What is less clear is whether the high levels of satisfaction are mirrored by good-quality analgesia. Studies comparing efficacy with intramuscular regimens have reported reduced opioid use, early hospital discharge and improved efficacy. Others have failed to demonstrate any improvement in pain scores, despite high levels of satisfaction.

It is important that when the technique is started (usually in recovery) or after interruptions (e.g. a blocked infusion) adequate loading doses are used to establish good analgesia.

Many anaesthetists consider PCA to be the optimum form of analgesia for major surgery, and the technique is generally popular with nurses.

SIDE-EFFECTS

All the side-effects attributable to opioids are possible when these drugs are used via PCA (see Chapter 3) **NB**: Nausea and vomiting are common, and may be reduced by the addition of an antiemetic (usually cyclizine or droperidol) to the drug reservoir.

Preoperative patient explanation is essential to maximize the technique's efficacy. Ideally, written material should be presented either before the patient reaches hospital or on the ward. Before surgery the patient should have further explanation and should be shown the handset.

Training of staff involved in the use of PCA will likewise improve the efficacy and safety of the technique. Regular involvement of a pain team should achieve this. Specific training may be a requirement before nurses can 'extend their role'.

MONITORING

Monitoring is essential to ensure the safety and utility of the technique. In a few hospitals PCA is restricted to high-dependency areas but in most this is unnecessary. Pain assessment (at rest and during appropriate activity) should be regular, at least hourly for the first few hours and after changes are made to the regimen. An assessment of side-effects should occur at the same time, including an assessment of sedation, respiratory depression and a specific enquiry about nausea or vomiting.

The device should be monitored to detect malfunction. Display settings should correspond with the prescription. Where patient demands and successes are displayed this may be noted. The syringe should be checked to confirm that the correct volume and no more has left the syringe.

ALTERNATIVES TO PCA AND MODIFICATIONS

Variable-dose PCA using a handset with three buttons corresponding to morphine boluses of 0.5, 1.0 and 1.5 mg has been reported to be successful. Patients rapidly learned which bolus size produced the effects they desired.

Target controlled infusions have been devised for short-acting agents such as alfentanil. An infusion based on a pharmacokinetic model and patient data is used to achieve a target blood concentration of the drug. Patient demands trigger an increase in the rate of infusion. If no patient demands are made within a fixed period infusion rate reduces.

EPIDURAL ANALGESIA

Epidural analgesia is used for postoperative pain management in most hospitals and its use has increased over the last decade. Its efficacy is not disputed, but its safety and risk – benefit ratio are widely discussed.

GENERAL CONSIDERATIONS

Epidural analgesia is frequently used for thoracic, abdominal and major vascular surgery. It is also suitable for pelvic and lower limb surgery. When epidural analgesia is planned it is normal to site the catheter immediately preoperatively and use epidural anaesthesia with or without general anaesthesia for surgery. An ideal block provides segmental analgesia corresponding only to those spinal segments from which pain is arising. Blocking of segments outside this area produces unnecessarily wide sympathetic block and motor weakness. Analgesia may be maintained by infusion or intermittent bolus. When an infusion is used, as is common, a combination of low-concentration local anaesthetic and opioid is suitable. Intermittent injections with long-acting opioids (diamorphine, morphine) are an alternative. After major surgery epidural analgesia is often continued for 48–72 hours. Where clinical indications exist it can be continued for much longer periods.

The pharmacology of spinally administered local anaesthetics and opioids is discussed in Chapter 2.

COMBINATIONS OF LOCAL ANAESTHETIC AND OPIOID

Neither local anaesthetics nor opioids provide ideal epidural analgesia when administered alone. When the two are combined analgesia is improved, and side-effects, many of which are dose dependent, are markedly reduced. Side-effects include nausea, vomiting, sedation, itch, urinary retention, respiratory depression, hypotension and muscle weakness. Complete analgesia with minimal side-effects may be achieved. Bupivacaine is the local anaesthetic most commonly used and can be reduced to concentrations below 0.1% when used in conjunction with an opioid. This produces minimal motor and limited proprioceptive block. Fentanyl (1–10 μg/ml) and diamorphine (50–200 μg/ml) are the opioids most commonly used with local anaesthetics.

CONTRAINDICATIONS TO USE OF EPIDURAL ANALGESIA

Absolute

- Patient refusal
- Inadequate facilities (to supervise, detect and treat complications)
- Allergy to intended agents.

Relative

Although each of these factors makes the use of epidural analgesia less safe, the risks of the technique must be balanced against the likely benefits for the individual. This is best discussed with each patient.

- Sepsis (local or generalized)
- Abnormality of clotting or platelet function
- Actual or potential severe haemorrhage
- Fixed cardiac output
- Spinal deformity
- Pre-existing or active neurological defect or disease.

ADVANTAGES AND DISADVANTAGES OF EPIDURAL ANALGESIA

The advantages of epidural analgesia are listed below. Where specific effects relate to epidural analgesia with local anaesthetic or with opioid the letters LA or O follow, respectively.

- Excellent analgesia is possible
- Unhindered movement, permitting physiotherapy, coughing and early mobilization
- Improved diaphragmatic function following abdominal and thoracic surgery (LA)
- Improved respiratory function following abdominal and thoracic surgery
- Reduced chest infections
- Reduced duration of ileus, leading to early enteral feeding (LA)
- Improved gastrointestinal perfusion
- Reduction in postoperative myocardial ischaemia by improving the oxygen delivery to demand ratio (LA)
- Improved graft preservation following vascular reconstruction
- Reduction in thromboembolic disease by improving arterial and venous blood flow, obtunding procoagulant changes following surgery, reducing platelet adhesiveness (LA) and allowing early mobilization
- Stress response to surgery reduced for some procedures (including reduced catecholamine levels, reduced levels of catabolic hormones and reduced insulin resistance). The clinical significance of this is unclear.
- Shorter stay in intensive care

These wide-ranging potential advantages must be carefully balanced against the disadvantages associated with the technique:

- Increased monitoring required to maintain safety
- Increased time spent in intensive care or high-dependency units if the technique is restricted to those sites
- Minor complications of the technique:
  - dural puncture with subsequent headache. Rates are quoted from 0.3 to 8% and are reduced by the use of saline to identify the epidural space and by use of the paramedian technique
  - backache (less of a problem than in the obstetric population)
  - catheter transection or knotting
- Complications of the use of spinal local anaesthetics
- Complications of the use of spinal opioids
- Masking of painful complications such as limb ischaemia.
- Neurological damage from bleeding, direct trauma or injection errors

Remember: Neurological damage (direct trauma, haematoma formation) is extremely rare. However, excessive motor blockade or severe backache should prompt careful neurological evaluation.

MONITORING

Monitoring should:

- assess analgesia
- detect side-effects (e.g. nausea and vomiting, mild hypotension)
- detect major complications (e.g. cord compression, severe hypotension).

Assessment of analgesia follows routine practice, as described elsewhere. Respiratory depression is most frequently monitored by means of respiratory rate, although this has limitations. Pulse oximetry is becoming more widely available on wards.

The epidural entry site should be inspected regularly for signs of catheter movement, infusate leakage or infection. Filters and connections should also be checked for leaks and disconnections.

The safety of epidural analgesia on general wards remains controversial despite reports of its safety when supervised by an acute pain service. The risks of severe hypotension and respiratory depression or arrest are lower with epidural analgesia than with intravenous opioid infusions if supervision is adequate.

CAUDAL ANALGESIA

The epidural space may be approached through the sacrococcygeal membrane. Blockade performed via this route is termed 'caudal blockade'. Caudal block is frequently used for supplementing general anaesthesia for perineal and lower abdominal surgery, particularly in children. A bolus of opioid can provide prolonged analgesia.

Caudal catheters may be inserted and prolonged blockade maintained. This is uncommon in adult practice as the epidural space can usually be entered at another site. Skin fixation and sterility are difficult to maintain.

PATIENT-CONTROLLED EPIDURAL ANALGESIA (PCEA)

This technique applies the principles of PCA to epidural analgesia. A reservoir of drug is administered in small boluses after patient demands. A lockout period provides a limit to the quantity of drug that may be used. A background infusion is more common with PCEA than with conventional PCA. Most research into PCEA has been in the field of obstetric analgesia. In that environment it produces high levels of satisfaction, good analgesia, and reduces the amount of drug administered. It has been less fully evaluated for postoperative analgesia.

INTRATHECAL ANALGESIA

Subarachnoid local anaesthetics provide excellent conditions for surgery but last only for a short period of time. The associated side-effects may be unpleasant (complete motor and sensory blockade). Unless an intrathecal catheter is inserted (see below) this method of analgesia is impractical for postoperative use.

Intrathecal opioids may provide longer-lasting analgesia than local anaesthetics. The duration of analgesia after a single dose of opioid is unpredictable and widely variable. Fentanyl and sufentanil may be effective for 1–6 hours. Morphine and diamorphine are effective for 4–24 hours, and occasionally for 48 hours. Side-effects are also unpredictable and are dose dependent. Common side-effects, as with epidural opioids, are nausea, itch, sedation and urinary retention. Observations to detect respiratory depression are mandatory for at least 12 hours after intrathecal morphine.

CONTINUOUS SUBARACHNOID ANALGESIA

The 'single-shot' intrathecal technique offers no advantage over epidural analgesia. The introduction of a very fine catheter (microspinal catheter) allows intermittent top-ups or infusion techniques to be used to maintain analgesia. Intrathecal catheter production has ceased in many countries and the popularity of the technique is declining.

POSTOPERATIVE PAIN MANAGEMENT IN SPECIAL CIRCUMSTANCES

DAY-CASE SURGERY

The principles of postoperative pain management for day-case surgery are no different from those used in other forms of surgery, but the emphasis is slightly different. Operations are selected so that pain can be expected to be controllable without potent opioids. Pain is anticipated and operative analgesia given to prevent it. Local analgesia is widely used for infiltration and nerve blockade. No wound is too small to be infiltrated. Plexus blockade and central blockade are rarely used, with the exception of caudal blockade. Local anaesthetic techniques should be selected to produce minimal motor and proprioceptive block in these ambulant patients. Paracetamol and NSAIDs are used whenever not contraindicated, and may be usefully given before surgery so that effective blood levels are established when surgery finishes. Balanced analgesia is frequently needed to provide adequate pain relief while avoiding side-effects that necessitate admission.

Immediate postoperative analgesic requirements should therefore be expected to be minimal. Oral weak opioid analgesia is used as required. If this is ineffective adjuncts may be used. If these also fail potent opioids should be considered. If potent opioids are necessary the patients should be carefully assessed to ensure admission is not warranted. Poorly controlled pain and significant side-effects of analgesia (especially nausea and vomiting) are indications for longer stay or overnight admission. Emetic sequelae during transport home are frequent after opioid analgesia, and are a common cause for admission. Antiemetics should be administered routinely with opioids.

Enough analgesics should be given to the patient to take home. A combination of a weak opioid/paracetamol and an NSAID is appropriate.

Unfortunately a large proportion of patients, including those with good pain relief in hospital, experience pain severe enough to warrant calling out their general practitioner in the first 24 hours after day surgery.

MANAGEMENT OF POSTOPERATIVE PAIN IN CHILDREN

Introduction

Children are given less analgesia than adults. They are given lower doses and greater intervals elapse between doses. Potent analgesia is given to children less frequently than to adults and minor analgesics are introduced at an early stage postoperatively.

All the reasons for poor pain management in adults apply to children, but there are others specific to children:

- A mistaken belief that small children do not experience pain, particularly neonates and infants
- A belief that if children do experience pain it is less severe than for adults
- Fears that side-effects of analgesics are more likely in children
- Difficulty in assessing pain in children
- Belief that children would prefer pain to an injection.

It is clear now that children of all ages experience pain and that adverse physiological responses accompany pain. There is no logical reason to assume that children's pain should be any less severe than that of an adult. Injections can often be avoided. It should rarely be necessary for a child to have more than a few analgesic injections, and modes of delivery that avoid injection should be considered.

The side-effects of analgesics may be problematic in very young infants and are discussed below. In appropriate doses the side-effects of most analgesics are less frequent than in the adult or elderly population. This is partly because the majority of children undergoing surgery are healthy and with good physiological reserve.

Paediatric doses of analgesics may be very small. Errors in calculation are frequent and may lead to serious consequences if a decimal point is misplaced. For those unfamiliar with paediatric dosing great care is needed, and calculations should be checked by more than one person.

When small doses are given the volume of drug administered may also be small. From an ampoule containing 10 mg/ml drawing up 0.02 ml (0.2 mg) is difficult and accuracy is unlikely. Diluting the drug to a larger volume increases accuracy, but may complicate calculations further. Diluting to 1 mg/ml is a good compromise. When the drug is given in a very small volume administered to a cannula with a side port it is important either to increase the volume further by dilution or to flush the cannula to ensure all the drug is delivered.

Consequences of poor pain management in children

- Adverse physiological effects (as in adults, see above)
- Adverse psychological effects.

The psychological consequences of poor pain management may be serious, particularly if pain is repeatedly undertreated and when children are given false information about painful procedures. The child's trust is lost and he or she may become anxious, fearful and uncooperative. Rational explanation then becomes impossible. The relationship between parent and child may also suffer.

PRINCIPLES OF PAIN MANAGEMENT IN CHILDREN

Many are the same as those that guide pain management in adults:

- Analgesia should be based on regular **assessment** of pain.
- Treatment should be **individualized** for each patient.
- Where pain can be **prevented** efforts should be made to achieve this.
- Side-effects must be kept to an acceptable minimum.
- **Balanced analgesia** may be used to improve efficacy and decrease side-effects.
- **Restoration of function** should be a clear goal.

In addition attention should be paid to:

- the differing psychological needs of children
- differing physiological development and reserve
- differing pharmacokinetics and pharmacodynamics
- specific complications in children.

ASSESSMENT OF PAIN IN CHILDREN (see also Chapter 9)

Pain assessment aims to detect pain, quantify its severity and assess the response to treatment. Quantifying pain is important so that initial treatment can be chosen and the response to that treatment determined.

As children become older this becomes progressively easier. Below the age at which children can rationalize, and especially below the verbal age, this is extremely difficult. Assessment often relies on objective measures to identify and quantify a subjective experience.

In young children crying may be a response to many causes of distress. Conversely a child may become immobile in a fearful attempt to avoid pain, and this may mimic a pain-free state. Pain may be hidden to avoid injections.

Methods to detect pain:

- Self-report from the child
- Report from an adult familiar with the child
- Interpretation of physiological alterations (e.g. respiratory rate, heart rate, pallor)
- Behavioural signals (e.g.: facial expression, posture, movement, guarding and protection of an injured site).

Self-report is the most reliable tool. Parental reporting and assessment is similar to clinician assessment but rates pain consistently higher. As observers generally underestimate pain this parental score probably reflects the child's pain better than the clinician's.

Scoring systems

Attempts to quantify pain have led to a variety of scoring systems. These should be easy to use, reliable and unequivocal. Results should be reproducible and validated on a wide population.

Beyond the pre-verbal age assessment based on words and pictures is helpful. A pictorial visual analogue can use images such as temperature on a thermometer, colours on a face, numbers or verbal descriptions. These are usually restricted to five levels or fewer. A pain ladder and a scale based on expressive faces are frequently used.

Acute pain services

It has become increasingly accepted that pain management in children is important and may be complicated. This is partly due to an increased general awareness of the inadequacies of pain management, and also because of the wider acceptance that small children and neonates feel pain and that this should be treated. This has led to the formation of paediatric acute pain services (APS) in a few large centres. In many smaller hospitals the adult APS will assist in the management of pain in children. There is some evidence that when such a service is established for children standards of pain management improve.

Methods of pain relief in children

The methods of pain relief in children are the same as those in adults. Minor alterations may be necessary.

Psychological

Psychological preparation and support during painful events is essential for children, as indicated above. Parental presence may be of more benefit than any other single measure. Parents can provide reassurance and distraction, reduce the depersonalization of the hospital environment, and reduce feelings of threat.

Sympathetic and caring treatment is a prerequisite for paediatric care. Communication should be directed to the child, at an appropriate level for them to understand.

Physical

Physical acts performed by parents or carers may provide pain relief. Cooling and rubbing are examples.

The environment where children are treated may markedly affect their response to pain. Efforts should be made to make the environment and the personnel non-threatening and child-friendly. Maintaining appropriate room temperature and avoiding prolonged starvation or dehydration are also important in preventing unnecessary distress.

Pharmacological

Opioids Potent opioids are necessary for both severe pain and some moderate pain. Morphine is the drug of choice and the preferred route is intravenous. Doses should be carefully titrated. If the intramuscular or subcutaneous route is used an indwelling cannula may be left in place to reduce the discomfort of injections. Subcutaneous infusions have been used. Opioid infusions are used more frequently than in adult practice to provide sustained plasma drug levels and analgesia.

Morphine in doses of **0.1–0.2 mg/kg** is appropriate, to be repeated until analgesia is achieved. Infusions of **0.01–0.03 mg/kg/h** may be used in appropriately monitored environments. These doses may be doubled for ventilated children. Bolus doses should be halved and infusion rates considerably reduced for neonates (e.g. **0.005–0.007 mg/kg/h**) because of altered pharmacokinetics.

Premature neonates are at risk of postoperative apnoeic episodes, the risk of which is increased by opioid analgesia. Opioid half-life is increased by hepatic immaturity. Low levels of α_1-glycoprotein increase the free fraction of drug. Opioid receptor subtypes may differ in affinity and sensitivity from those in the adult. Apnoea monitoring should be used until 50 weeks post-conceptual age. The use of local blocks where possible reduces this risk.

Morphine and fentanyl have prolonged elimination half-life in neonates. Morphine is metabolized to the sulphate rather than the glucuronide by the neonatal liver, and this alters potency.

PCA or nurse-controlled analgesia (with one identified proxy) may be used above 5 years of age. A background infusion is more frequently needed than in adult practice and may improve sleep. Although respiratory depression is rare, monitoring must be to the same standards as for adults. Appropriate bolus size is **0.02 mg/kg**, an infusion rate of **4 μg/kg/h** and a lockout period of **5 minutes**. PCA can be used by either the intravenous or the subcutaneous route.

Weak opioids Codeine is suitable for moderate pain in doses of 1–1.5 mg/kg.

Paracetamol Paracetamol is the most frequently used drug for postoperative analgesia in children. It is used in a dose of 15 mg/kg every 5 hours. It is effective in mild pain and is a useful adjunct for moderate or severe pain. Regular dosing and a preoperative dose improve efficacy. When used rectally the initial dose may need to be as high as 35 mg/kg. Elimination in infants is slower (2–5 hours) than in adults.

NSAIDs The use of NSAIDs in paediatric practice is increasing. Because of their immature renal function neonates clear NSAIDs slowly and half-life is increased. By 3 months of age pharmacokinetics are similar to those in adults.

Efficacy in infants has not been fully investigated. Similarly, the side-effect profile is poorly established. NSAIDs are effective analgesics and useful adjuncts to other forms of analgesia. Ibuprofen, diclofenac, mefenamic acid and ketorolac are popular.

Entonox This is a useful agent for short painful procedures in older children. It may be used for younger children but they need assistance. The operation of a demand valve, use of masks, unpleasant smell and nausea are all disadvantages.

Local anaesthesia Local anaesthesia provides excellent analgesia for children and may avoid the need for other analgesics completely. This is particularly the case after minor surgery (e.g. day surgery).

Several precautions are necessary:

- Relevant anatomy and landmarks differ from those in adults and in different age groups.
- Children tolerate the performance of local anaesthetic techniques less well than adults. This necessitates many blocks being performed during general anaesthesia. Some consider this reduces the safety of the technique.
- Toddlers with motor blockade may lack the understanding to limit efforts to walk, and injury is possible.

- Infant nerves are less myelinated and have smaller internodal distance than adults. Concentrations of local anaesthetics needed to block conduction are reduced and onset of blockade is fast.
- For a given dose of bupivacaine infants may have raised plasma levels. Metabolism of bupivacaine is reduced below 3 months. Safe doses are reduced. Recommended doses vary from 1 to 2.5 mg/kg bupivacaine.
- In neonates this problem is compounded: owing to reduced protein binding (low α-acid glycoprotein) and altered pH the free fraction of drug is increased in plasma. Drug elimination is impaired. The likelihood of adverse reaction therefore increases.

Topical EMLA and amethocaine gel are very suitable for painful venepuncture. They have little role in postoperative pain management but may be useful for circumcision. Topical local anaesthesia to the eye reduces pain after squint surgery.

Infiltration For minor surgery this can be the mainstay of analgesia for small incisions, such as many used in day-case surgery. Other analgesia may be reduced or eliminated. Restoration of function occurs early.

Nerve blocks Ilioinguinal blocks for groin surgery and penile blocks for penile surgery are commonly performed. Femoral blockade is also useful. Sciatic block may require high doses of local anaesthetic.

Caudal blockade This is the most frequently used block for children. It is suitable for subumbilical surgery. Large volumes of drug may provide analgesia for procedures above the umbilicus. Parents must be warned of potential motor blockade, and this may limit its use in day surgery. This is reduced by use of dilute local anaesthetics (e.g. 0.125% bupivacaine).

NB: In younger children the spinal cord and dural sac pass more caudally. In neonates the dural sac extends to S2 and may easily be entered during caudal injection. As ossification is not present in infants the S2/3 level can be used for epidural access.

Epidural catheters may be inserted at the caudal level. This may be technically easier than at other levels. A catheter may be passed as high as the thoracic level. Infection is uncommon. The catheter is then used for bolus injection of continuous infusion. The same standard of care and monitoring is required as for other epidural regimens. Caudal opioids and ketamine can provide prolonged analgesia, but increased postoperative monitoring is required.

Central blockade

Epidural analgesia This is becoming more widespread as experience and equipment have improved. The principles of epidural analgesia follow those of adult practice. Side-effects are similar, although hypotension is uncommon. The use of epidural infusions, particularly if they contain opioids, should be restricted to a specialized high-dependency unit and is rarely practised outside specialist centres.

CHANGING PRACTICE

More perioperative analgesia is now given to children – and particularly infants – than a decade ago. The use of local anaesthesia and paracetamol is widespread in all age groups. Opioid use remains restricted in preterm infants. The use of all classes of analgesic has increased, as has their combination in balanced analgesia. Central regional blockade for major surgery extending to very young children has also increased. The choice of analgesic method is still limited in some cases by lack of sufficient postoperative facilities.

CHAPTER 11

MANAGEMENT OF PAIN FOLLOWING TRAUMA

INTRODUCTION

A large casualty department may treat over 50 000 patients each year. A third of these will present with pain associated with trauma, the severity of which varies from trivial to life-threatening. Similarly the pain of trauma can be a minor inconvenience or all-consuming. The correlation between severity of injury and severity of pain is very poor and markedly affected by the circumstances of the injury. Several surveys have demonstrated that acute pain is treated poorly in casualty departments.

RESUSCITATION

Treatment of pain has a high priority but it is *not* the first priority. The presence of life-threatening or health-threatening injury must precede the treatment of pain. Resuscitation, with attention to the maintenance of a safe airway, cervical spine immobilization, restoration of breathing and circulation, is imperative.

SEVERITY OF INJURY

Minor injuries:

- Sprains
- Minor lacerations, abrasions, fractures and dislocations
- Minor scalds and burns
- Minor head injuries.

Intermediate injury:

- Larger lacerations, fractures and dislocations
- Larger scalds and burns
- Significant head injuries.

Major injury:

- Lacerations affecting major neurovascular tissues
- Fractures and dislocations of long bones, pelvis and chest
- Major scalds and burns (> 15% body surface area)
- Injuries affecting underlying viscera (chest, abdomen, pelvis)
- Major head injuries.

Analgesia should be addressed as soon as life-threatening injuries are treated. During this period, reassurance and explanation to patients (who may have considerably more fear than pain, despite severe injury) are vital.

Patients with intermediate trauma also need major injuries and hypovolaemia excluded and treated. Pain relief should be started while this secondary survey occurs.

For those with minor injuries pain may be the most significant part of the injury. Analgesia should be given early.

In almost all cases of pain due to injury the pain is **nociceptive**. The majority of cases involve somatic pain and this should be amenable to analgesics readily available in casualty. Fewer cases will be due to visceral nociceptive pain, and fewer still to neuropathic pain. These cases may be more difficult to treat.

ADEQUACY OF ANALGESIA IN THE A & E DEPARTMENT

Analgesia in the emergency department is frequently inadequate: up to 60% of patients presenting to casualty with pain receive no analgesia. When analgesia is administered this is often after considerable delay and by inappropriate routes in inadequate doses. Children presenting with pain are particularly poorly managed in this respect. When painful procedures are performed analgesia is often inadequate or absent.

Contributory reasons for this are:

- Observers consistently underestimate patients' pain
- Appropriate delay to exclude and treat major injury
- Inappropriate delay from slow onset of analgesia: too little, given infrequently, by the wrong route (e.g. i.m., s.c.)
- Fear of general effects of analgesia (e.g. sedation in head injuries)
- Fear of specific side-effects of analgesia (particularly respiratory depression from opioids)
- Fear of masking clinical signs.

Analgesia should be rapidly effective with minimal side-effects. No drugs currently available are without side-effects, and these must be taken into account in further evaluation of the patient. Changes in vital signs after analgesia should be critically evaluated rather than attributed to analgesia. The need for careful monitoring of patients in the first hours following major injury cannot be overemphasized.

Pain in the injured patient has a number of physiological and other sequelae:

- Raised catecholamine levels
- Tachycardia, hypertension, vasoconstriction
- Hyperventilation, dehydration and exhaustion
- Gastric stasis and increased gastric acidity
- Nausea and vomiting
- Sensitization of peripheral and central nervous system
- Loss of confidence in carers
- Inability to communicate with carers.

The advantages of adequate analgesia are:

- humanitarian
- maintenance of cooperation
- maintenance of therapeutic relationship
- reduction in adverse physiological sequelae
- avoidance of psychological sequelae.

ANALGESIA AND CLINICAL SIGNS

Fear of masking clinical signs is one of the most important misconceptions underlying inadequate analgesic provision in the emergency department. Effective analgesia improves patient cooperation and so can aid diagnosis.

There is no evidence that adequate pain relief causes diagnostic confusion.

HEAD INJURIES

Head injury cases that warrant admission require neurological observations but the patient may have pain from the head injury itself or from injuries elsewhere. Local anaesthetic techniques are sensible wherever possible for associated injuries, as central neurological signs will not be affected. Potent opioids are traditionally avoided. Paracetamol is an effective mild analgesic and adjunct. Codeine is traditionally favoured as it causes minimal sedation and less pupillary constriction or respiratory depression than potent opioids, although its efficacy is questionable.

Patients with minor head injuries that are allowed home should not be given sedating analgesics. Carers at home will not be able to distinguish drug-induced from injury-induced sedation.

OVERVIEW OF ANALGESIC MODALITIES

There are many approaches to pain relief in trauma. For optimum analgesia methods from each group should be used together. All facets are important, and neglect in any one may lead to inadequate analgesia. Useful modes of pain relief are outlined in Table 11.1

TABLE 11.1 Methods of pain relief in trauma

Method	*Examples*
Physical	Surface cooling of burns Splinting fractures Reducing dislocations
Pharmacological – systemic	Opioids NSAID Ketamine Entonox General anaesthesia
Pharmacological – local	Topical Infiltration Nerve blocks Regional or plexus blocks
Psychological	Information and explanation Reassurance Emotional support Behavioural methods

PHYSICAL

These form part of first aid and may have been performed before the patient arrives in A&E.

Reduction of fractures may be exceedingly painful, and the analgesia required to achieve sufficient pain relief may lead to side-effects after reduction. A brief general anaesthetic is safer than heavy, inadequate sedation and should not delay discharge excessively.

PHARMACOLOGICAL – SYSTEMIC

Opioids

Potent opioids

Opioids are the mainstay of analgesia in acute pain. In order to be rapidly effective they must be given intravenously, as the intramuscular (and subcutaneous) routes have several disadvantages:

- Slow onset
- Variable onset
- Altered bioavailablity in repeated doses at the same site (e.g. pethidine)
- Very poor absorption in conditions of poor peripheral perfusion, such as blood loss, hypothermia and fear, all of which are common in trauma. Inadequate pain relief following i.m. analgesia may be followed by resuscitation and further analgesia. Improved perfusion and absorption may then produce effective overdosage.

Advantages of opioids in trauma

- Good efficacy
- Rapid onset if given intravenously
- Few absolute contraindications
- Readily available.

Disadvantages of opioids in trauma

- Sedation is an important side-effect of opioids. Adequate analgesia should not require excessive sedation. Sedation increases the likelihood of airway obstruction, significant respiratory depression and hypoxia. Sedation following analgesia must *not* be assumed to be drug induced.
- Nausea and vomiting are common, particularly with first doses of opioids. An antiemetic should be given routinely
- Respiratory depression is usually mild and is at a maximum within 10 minutes of i.v. administration. It is delayed with i.m. injections. This does have implications for those with chest, head or other major injury. Monitoring is essential, although respiratory rate is an unreliable index. Hypoxia can be prevented by administering additional oxygen.
- Pupillary constriction necessitates caution in assessment of the head-injured patient.
- Dysphoria and confusion.
- Short or intermediate duration.

Morphine given intravenously has peak effect within 5 minutes. This is also true for pethidine and diamorphine. An estimated loading dose should be given, taking into account the patient's age, size, general condition and injuries. An initial dose of 5 mg morphine in an adult is a guide. The patient should be attended and pain, sedation and respiration monitored constantly for 5 minutes. If analgesia is inadequate, in the absence of important side-effects further analgesia should be given after 3–5 minutes. Increments (1–3 mg of morphine) are given in this manner until good analgesia is achieved without major side-effects.

Minor opioids

Codeine, dihydrocodeine and dextropropoxyphene are all weak opioids. They may be given orally and are often combined with paracetamol, which increases their efficacy. Codeine and dihydrocodeine may also be given by injection, and are favoured for in-patients with head injuries (see above).

Weak receptor affinity limits the analgesic efficacy of codeine, dihydrocodeine and dextropropoxyphene. Constipation and nausea can be particular problems.

Oral analgesia is appropriate for patients with minor injuries being discharged. For more serious injury the gastric stasis produced by pain and severe injury makes oral drugs inappropriate.

Partial agonists

Partial agonists may have a marginally greater safety profile than potent opioids. For this reason they are frequently used before arrival in hospital. However, analgesia is poor and they decrease the efficacy of subsequently administered full agonist opioids.

Tramadol Has dual analgesic actions (opioid and non-opioid) and is reported to have a low risk of respiratory depression. It is effective in moderate pain. It may be given orally or i.m./i.v. Reports of efficacy are conflicting and nausea and vomiting are common. There have been reports of convulsions, dependence and withdrawal following its use. It is not a controlled drug.

Non-steroidal anti-inflammatory drugs (NSAIDs)

This class of drugs is probably underused in casualty departments. They are effective alone for minor pain and are effective adjuncts in moderate or severe pain. Side-effects are uncommon when the drugs are used for the short periods likely after trauma. However, where contraindications such as asthma, peptic ulcer disease or renal impairment exist the drugs should be avoided, particularly in the elderly. New agents and routes of administration have introduced more possibilities for their use.

Advantages of NSAIDs in trauma

- Effective analgesia in mild to moderate pain
- Opioid-sparing effect in severe pain
- Minimal effect on vital signs
- No risk of sedation or respiratory depression
- Long duration of action
- Available by several routes.

Disadvantages of NSAIDs in trauma

- Side-effects may make them unsuitable for a proportion of patients
- Inadequate analgesia in severe pain
- Delay in onset of analgesia, even when given intravenously
- Potential risk of bleeding in major trauma
- Potential for peptic ulceration in major trauma
- Potential for impaired renal blood flow in hypovolaemia.

Paracetamol

Though widely used this may not be used to its maximal effect. It is the drug of choice for minor injury owing to its low side-effect profile in therapeutic dosage. It has a useful antipyretic function. Analgesia may be improved by the addition of a weak opioid or NSAID. Side-effects will rise with the improved analgesia.

Dosage in adults is 4 g/day and it is more effective when given regularly. Children may be prescribed 15 mg/kg every 5 hours; 35 mg/kg may be necessary as an initial dose if it is given rectally.

Inhalational analgesia

Entonox is a mixture of 50% nitrous oxide in oxygen (see Chapter 13). It is a potent analgesic and is available in some ambulances and most casualty departments. Up to 10% of patients derive no benefit from it. Side-effects include nausea and vomiting (5%), vertigo (20%) and drowsiness (50%).

Advantages of entonox in trauma
- Good analgesia
- Rapid onset of effect (less than 60 seconds)
- Rapid cessation of effect
- Minimal 'hangover' of effects
- Raises inspired oxygen fraction (to 0.5).

Disadvantages of entonox in trauma
- Expands air-filled spaces (see below)
- Requires patient understanding, effort and co-operation to be effective
- May not be tolerated because of sedation, lightheadedness or nausea
- May raise intracranial pressure in severe head injury
- Requires scavenging to protect staff members.

Entonox is particularly useful for brief painful procedures, such as the application of dressings. It may also be used to augment other forms of analgesia, e.g. for manipulation of minor dislocations. If it is ineffective general anaesthesia may well be required.

Owing to its low solubility in blood nitrous oxide diffuses into gas-filled cavities. In acute trauma this may cause significant problems: conversion of a simple pneumothorax into a tension pneumothorax is most frequently quoted. Other potential problems include pneumoperitoneum and pneumocephalus following abdominal and head injury respectively. Entonox should therefore not be used in chest, abdominal or head injury until full evaluation has been made.

Ketamine

This anaesthetic agent has been advocated for analgesia in trauma. It is used extensively 'in the field'. It produces a state of profound analgesia with apparent superficial sleep: 'dissociative anaesthesia'. It may be used in doses of 0.5 mg/kg i.v. and is effective after approximately 1–2 minutes, lasting up to 10 minutes. Given i.m. in doses of 1–3 mg/kg dissociation occurs after 2–10 minutes and lasts longer. Its reputation for safety arises because it is the only anaesthetic agent to stimulate respiration and has a limited effect on laryngeal reflexes.

Advantages of ketamine in trauma

- Profound analgesia with maintenance of consciousness
- Limited effects on ventilation or laryngeal reflexes
- α-Adrenergic agonism maintains blood pressure
- Bronchodilation
- May be used 'in the field', for instance during extraction from vehicles.

Disadvantages of ketamine in trauma

- Airway maintenance cannot be guaranteed
- Hypertension and tachycardia
- Muscular rigidity may impede manipulation of dislocations and fractures
- Increased salivation (reduced by atropine premedication)
- Direct myocardial depression may rarely lead to collapse in patients with maximal sympathetic drive
- Emergence phenomena (agitation and restlessness) and vivid (often highly unpleasant) dreams up to 24 hours later.

LOCAL ANAESTHESIA

Local anaesthesia can be very effective, safe and economical. Expertise and facilities for resuscitation must be available if major total anaesthesia techniques are used. Commonly used techniques are summarized in Table 11.2.

TABLE 11.2 Local anaesthetic techniques in trauma

Local anaesthetic technique	*Uses*
Topical	Prior to venepuncture in children Anaesthesia of mucous membranes
Local infiltration	Suturing Analgesia for lacerations Fracture haematoma infiltration
Intravenous regional analgesia	Reduction of forearm fractures
Nerve block	Femoral nerve block for femur fractures Intercostal block for single rib fractures
Plexus block	Brachial plexus block for forearm fractures Lumbar plexus block for femur fractures
Regional block	Thoracic epidural for multiple rib fractures

Advantages of local anaesthesia in trauma

- Negligible systemic side-effects in safe dosage
- Rapid onset of infiltration and single nerve blocks
- Muscular relaxation for limb manipulation
- Avoidance of side-effects of opioids and NSAIDs.

The avoidance of sedation and respiratory depression in the severely injured is a particularly useful effect of local anaesthetic analgesia.

Disadvantages of local anaesthesia in trauma

- Infiltration itself is painful
- Local anaesthesia may be ineffective at sites of inflammation as tissue acidosis impedes nerve penetration
- Blocks may be time-consuming to administer
- Skill and specialist techniques may be required for some blocks
- Difficult with children
- Adrenaline must be avoided for end arteries (e.g. digits, ears, penis)
- Intense analgesia may mask clinical signs (e.g. compartment syndrome)
- There is a small potential for life-threatening complications.

Careful observation is needed to detect the signs of compartment syndrome in a patient with an effective plexus or regional block.

PSYCHOLOGICAL APPROACHES

Injury is frequently unexpected. The injured patient is rapidly propelled into an unfamiliar atmosphere over which they have little or no control. Pain may be considerably modified by the circumstances of injury. Fear and anxiety of the uncertain future, over others involved in an accident and mundane concerns may exacerbate pain.

Explanation and accurate information will help most patients. Truthful reassurance contributes to alleviation of anxiety and can reduce pain. Concentration on positive thoughts may help as distraction or morale boosting. Even simple tasks such as passing information to work or family may have beneficial effects. The presence of relatives at an appropriate time during resuscitation is advocated by several sources.

Injury is a particularly unpleasant experience for children and this may be magnified by parental distress. Parental involvement may provide essential support, reduce anxiety and give effective distraction for both parties.

CHOICE OF ANALGESIA

The choice of analgesia often depends on several factors, which include the severity of the injury and whether the patient is to be admitted or not. All forms of analgesia may be used for those being admitted. Effective methods with the potential for side-effects are acceptable, providing monitoring is sufficient to detect them and treatment is available should they occur.

For those to be discharged home a limited variety of interventional analgesia is available. Medication should have a low incidence of side-effects and these must not be serious. Potent opioids should not be used and local anaesthetic techniques that produce significant motor weakness, altered proprioception or sensory loss must be used with extreme caution. Consideration should be given as to whether analgesia will be adequate after drugs administered in hospital wear off. Combination therapy may be possible: for example, analgesia may start with local anaesthesia administered at the hospital and the patient may be sent home with paracetamol to be taken regularly, and an NSAID, weak opioid or both to add if analgesia is inadequate. Advice should routinely be given on important side-effects and what to do should these occur.

CHAPTER 12

MANAGEMENT OF PAIN FOLLOWING BURNS

INTRODUCTION

Almost all patients with cutaneous burns experience pain, and this is often prolonged and severe. Pain is usually associated with considerable distress and psychological sequelae are common. Burn victims do not always feel pain at or immediately after the time of injury, as pain may be inhibited by other activities essential to survival. Patients with severe burns will require acute medical intervention, including airway management and fluid resuscitation, but analgesia must be given at the same time. Patients who are burned less severely may have pain as their main complaint. Pain management in burned patients tends to be inadequate. Patients may have pain for a number of reasons:

- From the burn injury itself. This is felt at the site of the injury and in the surrounding tissues. The pain is constant and exacerbated by movement, including medical examination and, occasionally, breathing. In partial-thickness burns nerve endings are damaged but continue to function. There is local release of the mediators of inflammation, which causes pain. Full-thickness burns cause greater damage to nerve endings and pain from the site of thermal injury may be less than with partial-thickness burns. However, full-thickness burns are often surrounded by areas of partial-thickness burns. Thermal injury is often associated with peripheral and central hyperexcitability (see Chapters 1 and 19), which enhances the pain experience.
- Pain related to burn therapy. Burns patients undergo multiple therapeutic procedures during their hospital stay. Repeated changes of dressings are necessary, and are associated with severe pain. Other therapeutic interventions, such as wound debridement, are painful and skin grafting, despite improving pain in the burned area, may result in pain at the donor site. Pain may also arise from other measures involved in management of the sick patient, e.g. nasogastric and tracheal intubation, urinary catheters and intravenous cannulae. Physiotherapy, especially in the early stages, is likely to be painful.
- Pain during tissue healing. Regeneration of damaged nerve endings causes pain. Patients may also experience other unpleasant sensory phenomena, such as itching and paraesthesiae. The development of scars or contractures may be painful.

ASSESSMENT OF PAIN

Assessment of burns pain by doctors and nurses is notoriously unsatisfactory. Severely burned patients may be unable to report their experience of pain, particularly those who are mechanically ventilated. Patients with burned limbs may have difficulty in filling in visual analogue scales: verbal rating scales may be more useful. Patients can also be assessed with the McGill Pain Questionnaire as well as scales for anxiety, depression and other psychological sequelae of burns.

PSYCHOLOGICAL SEQUELAE OF BURNS

Burn patients may show fear, anxiety, depression and acute grief reactions. All of these will influence their experience of pain. High levels of anxiety appear to influence pain at rest more than that resulting from therapeutic procedures. Depression and anxiety become more prominent the longer the hospital stay, and it is therefore logical to provide psychological intervention early in the course of the patient's treatment. The psychological response may be appropriate to the injury or may develop into frank psychiatric disturbance.

METHODS OF PAIN RELIEF

These are summarized in Table 12.1.

The pain of burns varies greatly from patient to patient and treatment must be individualized. In addition, the pain experience for a single patient will fluctuate markedly during treatment and recovery, so pain must be continually reassessed and appropriate adjustments made to therapy.

TABLE 12.1 Pain therapy following burns

Method	*Comments*
Local therapy	
Cooling of burn with water	Useful in immediate post-burn period. Unsafe in electrical burns. Prolonged application can cause hypothermia
Application of dressings	Useful in immediate post-burn period
Surgical debridement and skin grafting	Can minimize pain in early post-burn period
Opioid drugs	Mainstay of analgesic management. Underadministered because of (erroneous) fears of addiction. Tolerance may develop when given for long periods to burn patients
i.v. infusion	Infusions usually set at predetermined rate and altered by nursing staff as necessary – problems because of wide variability in patient requirements and unreliability of assessment. Easy to give incremental doses prior to and during painful procedures.
PCA	Allows appropriate dose titration vs. patient needs. Not appropriate for young children or in the severely ill.
i.m and s.c.	Unsuitable in early post-burn period because may be reduced skin and muscle blood flow, leading to unpredictability in absorption. More suitable in later recovery stages
Oral	Useful after initial post-burn period. Sustained relief preparations may provide useful background analgesia or liquid morphine useful prior to painful procedures
Entonox	Useful for painful therapeutic procedures and physiotherapy. Rapid onset and offset of analgesia. Bone marrow depression is a problem of long-term administration – not known to what extent repeated short-term administration is a problem.
Local anaesthetic techniques	
Topical application	Topical lignocaine described in acute management of partial-thickness burns. EMLA used for split-skin grafting
Nerve blocks/regional blocks	Have been used as immediate analgesic therapy and before and after graft procedures. Considerable worries relating to introduction of infection – must only be used with rigorous aseptic technique
NSAIDS and paracetamol	Useful in later recovery phase. Should be avoided in patients with renal dysfunction
Psychological management	
Stress reduction, behavioural modification	Some promising results showing improvement in pain scores, analgesic consumption, anxiety, sense of control
Hypnosis, relaxation training, desensitization, individual psychotherapy	Reportedly successful but methodologically rigorous trials lacking

CHAPTER 13

OBSTETRIC ANALGESIA

INTRODUCTION

The pain of labour has been described as the most severe pain that most women will experience in their life. Around 80% of primiparous parturients rated the pain of labour before pain relief as severe or unbearable.

WHY IS OBSTETRIC PAIN 'SPECIAL'?

- It is prepared for to an extent far exceeding other causes of painful hospital admission.
- The painful process (labour) has a goal and a conclusion (delivery of the baby), unlike many other pains.
- There may be a feeling of personal challenge or fulfilment to the individual to endure labour without intervention. Some believe the pain is an essential part of whole birth process: this leads to or develops from social, cultural and peer pressure.
- Labour pain is considered 'normal' and regarded differently from other forms of acute pain.
- It is probably the most painful event in most women's lives.
- It is often worse than expected, and prolonged, especially in primiparae, which may lead to loss of confidence and emotional distress.

WHY IS IT IMPORTANT TO TREAT PAIN?

There are two principles:

- There is no known benefit of labour pain for either mother or fetus.
- Pain can produce adverse effects in both mother and fetus, which are summarized in Table 13.1.

Despite a large number of studies there is no consensus on the effect of analgesia on the progress of labour.

Pain management in labour should fulfil the following aims:

- No effect on maternal consciousness, alertness and cooperation
- No adverse maternal effects
- No effect on the progress of labour
- Maintenance of placental blood flow
- Minimal fetal and neonatal drug-induced depression.

TABLE 13.1 Adverse effects of pain on mother and fetus

Physiological effect	*Effect on mother*	*Effect on fetus*
Increased basal metabolic rate	Increased oxygen requirements	Reduced fetal oxygenation
Increased oxygen requirements Hyperventilation	Respiratory alkalosis and dehydration, intermittent apnoea and hypoxia (compounded by low functional residual capacity and sedative drugs)	Reduced fetal oxygenation (mechanism unclear, possible mechanical effect leads to reduced placental oxygen transfer)
Tachycardia, hypertension	Cardiovascular decompensation with severe cardiovascular disease (note elderly mothers) Risks for anaesthesia	Reduced placental blood flow, fetal acidosis
Hyperglycaemia and increased fatty acids	Ketone bodies Acidosis	Fetal acidosis
Increased catecholamines (and ACTH, ADH, cortisol)	Vasoconstriction and cardiovascular stimulation (pregnancy induced hypertension, risk of hypertensive surges) Increased oxygen utilisation Impaired uterine contraction Risks for anaesthesia	Reduced placental blood flow Fetal acidosis
Progressive increase in metabolic acidosis (hypoxia, catecholamines, dehydration)	Metabolic acidosis	Fetal acidosis
Increased gastrin release due to catecholamines Nausea and vomiting	Gastric stasis and increased acidity Increased risks with general anaesthetic	
Psychological	Anxiety, fear, panic, loss of control and cooperation Treatment causing amnesia, sedation, dissociation, depersonalization	

ACTH, adrenocorticotrophic hormone; ADH, antidiuretic hormone

MECHANISMS OF PAIN IN LABOUR

The structures contributing to pain in labour are summarized in Table 13.2.

METHODS OF PAIN RELIEF

These can be divided into:

- preparation of the patient
- Transcutaneous nerve stimulation
- inhalational analgesia
- systemic analgesia
- regional analgesia.

PREPARATION OF PATIENT

Antenatal education plays a major role in facilitating adequate analgesia by preparing the parturient for the pain of labour. This is only achieved if accurate information is provided regarding the nature and severity of labour pain, the methods of pain relief available and their proven efficacy. Antenatal classes should state which analgesic methods are and are not available in the local unit. Antenatal education about the painful nature of labour forms part of psychological preparation (psychoprophylaxis).

A supportive environment, with the presence of a partner or friend and the support provided by the relationship with a competent and empathetic midwife, has been shown to have considerable influence on analgesic requirements.

Relaxation techniques, such as 'breathing exercises', massage and hydrotherapy, have the major advantage of having no side-effects. These relaxation-based-techniques increase the ability to cope with pain (and may therefore reduce the need for other analgesic methods). It is unclear whether they have a true analgesic effect themselves.

Acupuncture and hypnosis are not widely available and are used by less than 0.5% of parturients. Although they are effective for both labour analgesia and operative delivery in suitably prepared self selected subjects, the techniques tend to be time-consuming and therefore costly.

TRANSCUTANEOUS NERVE STIMULATION (TENS)

The physiological basis for the efficacy of TENS is discussed in Chapter 8.

Pads are placed on the back over T10–L1 and the frequency and intensity of stimulation adjusted to maximize analgesia. TENS is available in more than half of UK obstetric units and is popular with labouring mothers. It is used by about 5% of parturients (usually in the early first stage), although its efficacy is unproven. It may postpone requirements for other analgesic interventions.

TABLE 13.2 Structures contributing to pain in labour

Stage of labour	*Structures and mechanisms*	*Site of referral*	*Anatomical organization*
First stage	Visceral uterine pain Contractions under isometric conditions Dilatation of cervix and lower segment retraction	Hypogastrium Back Bowel	Early T11–12 Later T10–L1 Nociceptive input from cervix/uterus via Aδ and C primary afferents Accompany nerves leaving lower thoracic/upper lumbar sympathetic chain
	Stretching and tearing of birth canal	Rectum, lower sacrum and anus, sometimes thighs	As second stage
Second and third stages	Vaginal and perineal pain Visceral and somatic Distension, tearing and cutting	Perineum, including vagina, rectum and anus	Presenting part presses on and distends pain-sensitive structures in the pelvis Pudendal nerve S2–4
Instrumental delivery	Uterine, vaginal and perineal pain Visceral and somatic Traction tearing and cutting	Perineum including, vagina, rectum and anus Abdomen and back	Principally as for second stage (sacral nerves) Involves more cephalad innervation if forceps enter uterus – T10 and downwards

INHALATIONAL ANALGESIA

At present nitrous oxide is the only widely available inhalational agent for analgesia in labour.

Nitrous oxide is a colourless and nearly odourless gas. Entonox is a mixture of 50% oxygen and 50% nitrous oxide. It is available in nearly all obstetric units and is suitable for use in the community. Its short-term use is generally acceptable to patients and there are few immediate side-effects. Problems that may occur include dizziness, dysphoria, loss of cooperation and nausea.

The delivery unit can be a tight-fitting mask or a mouthpiece. Only the woman should operate or hold the device, to prevent continued administration if excessive sedation occurs.

The analgesic effect of nitrous oxide is not instantaneous: maximum analgesia occurs after 45–60 seconds. It is important to instruct the mother to start using entonox as soon as her contraction begins and to stop when the contraction passes its peak. The agent's short duration allows rapid recovery between contractions. Hyperventilation of dry gas may lead to dry mouth, peripheral tingling (tetany), respiratory alkalosis and intermittent apnoea.

Entonox is used by up to 70% of women at some stage of labour. When it is used correctly up to 50% of parturients report satisfaction, and 17% slight pain relief. A third of women report no pain relief.

SYSTEMIC OPIOID THERAPY

Opioids were introduced to obstetric practice early this century and remain in widespread use. The pharmacology of the opioids has been discussed in Chapter 3.

The side-effects of opioids relevant to labour include:

- gastric stasis
- nausea and vomiting
- sedation
- fetal respiratory depression.

Route of administration

- Intramuscular. Although this is the most widely used route it is characterized by slow onset of effect (up to 1 hour) and therefore poor efficacy, particularly if used in response to pain rather than to prevent it. Bioavailablility may vary after repeated injections in the same site.
- Intravenous. This route provides rapid effect and bypasses bioavailability problems. It is therefore the most titratable method. One useful method is to give up to 20% of a planned dose every 2–5 minutes until the parturient is comfortable. Analgesia can then be prolonged with midwife- or patient-controlled infusion or bolus administration.

- Patient-controlled analgesia (PCA). This method was introduced in 1976 for the management of labour pain, but is more commonly used postoperatively.

Choice of drug

The pain of labour is poorly opioid sensitive. It has been reported that systemic opioids produce sedation and relaxation, but no reduction in pain scores. There is little to choose between drugs with respect to side-effects when given in equianalgesic doses.

Pethidine

Up to 40% of parturients receive pethidine during labour. Currently midwives can administer up to 200 mg in divided doses without a doctor's prescription. Problems include:

- It is highly sedating and emetic
- Repeated i.m. doses show markedly variable absorption and bioavailability
- Norpethidine, an active metabolite, decreases the seizure threshold (avoid in pregnancy-induced hypertension) and has a long half-life in the fetus
- Its use is associated with reduced fetal heart beat to beat variability.

Pethidine-induced respiratory depression in the neonate is readily reversed by naloxone.

Diamorphine

This is commonly used in Scotland. The drug must be prescribed by a doctor, which makes it less convenient for midwives. Whether there are increased or decreased risks to the neonate has not been determined by adequate trials.

REGIONAL ANALGESIA (Table 13.3)

TABLE 13.3 Regional anaesthetic techniques used in obstetrics

Regional technique	*Stage of labour*	*Comment*
Epidural	1st and 2nd	Commonest form of regional analgesia in labour
Spinal	1st and 2nd	Uncommon in labour, common for caesarian
Combined spinal–epidural	1st and 2nd	Extensively used in some centres
Caudal	2nd	Uncommon, not very effective: patchy block with risk of toxicity with high doses of LA
Pudendal	2nd	Common (by obstetrician) for vaginal analgesia
Paracervical	1st and 2nd	Rare in UK
Local infiltration	Delivery	Common, midwife or obstetrician administered

Epidural analgesia

This is regarded by many as the gold standard for labour analgesia. The potential side-effects are considerable but mostly avoidable.

Efficacy of epidural analgesia

Excellent analgesia is provided in more than 80% of cases and it is satisfactory in a further 10%. Pain scores are reduced by an average of more than 80%. Epidural analgesia is used in approximately 20% of labours. Variation between units is wide, from less than 5% to more than 50%. Up to a quarter of obstetric units have no provision for epidural analgesia.

Epidural analgesia is not universally accepted because of the side-effects. These may be trivial or, occasionally, life-threatening.

Epidural analgesia for the first stage of labour requires segmental analgesia, initially between dermatomes T11 and T12. This progresses as labour advances, and the second stage may require it to extend from T10 to S4.

Indications and contraindications (Table 13.4)

TABLE 13.4 Indications and contraindications to epidural analgesia

Indications	*Contraindications (all tend to be relative)*
Labour factors	Maternal refusal
Maternal request for analgesia	Inadequate skill
Complicated labour	Inadequate facilities
	Allergy to intended agents
	Sepsis (local or generalized)
Maternal factors	Coagulopathy
Coexisting medical disease	Severe haemorrhage,
Obstetric complications	Hypovolaemia
	Fixed cardiac output (cardiac disease)
Fetal factors	
Breech presentation	
Prematurity or intrauterine growth	
Retardation, chronic placental insufficiency	
Multiple pregnancy	
Fetal distress	

The principal benefits of epidural analgesia are:

- Very good analgesia
- Can be extended for operative delivery (thus avoiding risks of general anaesthesia)
- Beneficial to fetus in situations of uteroplacental insufficiency.

Adverse effects:

- Loss of awareness of contractions/birth
- Numbness and paraesthesiae
- Hypotension
- Retention or bladder distension requiring catheterization
- Shivering (central local anaesthetic toxicity or altered temperature regulation effect)
- Possibility of increased interventions – catheter, episiotomy
- Transient or permanent neurological sequelae.

Common and important problems

- **Hypotension** occurs in about 5% of labouring women after epidural analgesia. Dehydration and a reduction in sympathetic outflow with good pain relief may contribute. Aortocaval occlusion must be sought and corrected.
- **Dural puncture** occurs in between 0.5 and 2% of cases. Parturients should be warned of this. In 70% of cases where dural puncture with a Tuohy needle is recognized a positional headache requiring intervention develops.
- **Unrecognized subarachnoid or 'total spinal' anaesthesia**. These are rare events but potentially fatal in their effects.
- **Subdural placement** occurs when the catheter passes through the dura but not through the arachnoid mater. There may be marked hypotension.
- **Intravascular injection** is possible at insertion of the epidural and through subsequent migration of the catheter into a vein or artery. The danger if intravascular injection occurs is reduced by using small bolus injections or a continuous infusion.
- **Ineffective blockade** may be due to unilateral or absent block or missed segments.

> ***Backache*** **occurs in up to 45% of women after labour. It is unlikely that there is any relationship to epidural analgesia.**

There is a continuing trend towards the use of decreased concentrations of local anaesthetic in combination with opioids to minimize motor block and other undesirable side-effects of epidural and spinal analgesia. Controversy persists about the advantages of intermittent top-ups of analgesic agent compared to continuous infusion. Patient-controlled epidural analgesia has not gained widespread popularity.

Drugs used to provide epidural analgesia

Local anaesthetics. These can provide good analgesia but when used alone cause significant side-effects. Lower concentrations can be used effectively by combining local anaesthetics with opioids. Reducing motor blockade improves maternal satisfaction, reduces recumbency and the problems of nursing the immobile patient. Backache is also reduced.

Although a number of local anaesthetics have been used for pain relief in labour bupivacaine is the drug of choice, as it is long-acting, stable and has some sensory selectivity. Concentrations between 0.5 and 0.015% have been used: 0.5% produces full motor block and is sufficient for operative delivery. Higher concentrations can produce toxicity. Concentrations below 0.125% require other agents to provide good analgesia.

Opioids. These have the advantage of minimal sensory, motor and sympathetic blockade. The shivering seen with local anaesthetics is reduced. Opioid epidural analgesia is effective in early labour but inadequate alone in late first stage and second stage. Opioids are almost exclusively used in combination with local anaesthetics.

Fentanyl is the most commonly used drug. Boluses are between 25 and 100 μg and infusion rate between 8 and 40 μg/h. A bolus of 50–100 μg provides good analgesia in the first stage of labour. Onset is between 5 and 20 minutes and duration is up to 90 minutes. Boluses above 50 μg and infusion rates above 20 μg/h may delay gastric emptying. Cumulative doses up to 200 μg have little effect-on neonatal neurobehavioural scores, but larger doses may.

A combined bolus of local anaesthetic with opioid has rapid onset, better analgesia and more prolonged effect than either agent alone. This synergy is utilized by combining the agents as either bolus or infusion.

Advantages of spinal opioids include:

- incidence of missed segments and poor perineal analgesia is reduced
- hypotension, numbness, leg weakness and shivering are reduced
- mobility improved which may allow ambulation
- maternal satisfaction is improved
- low-dose infusions can be maintained throughout the second stage without interfering with maternal efforts to push.

Ambulatory epidurals. The use of epidural mixtures containing an opioid and a low-dose local anaesthetic can result in minimal loss of motor power and proprioception. Ambulation is often achieved by combining a subarachnoid block with an epidural (see below). Ambulation during labour has been said to hasten fetal descent and reduce aortocaval compression. Maternal satisfaction is improved. Comparisons between labour in the recumbent and the upright position supports the latter being shorter, less painful and preferred by mothers.

COMBINED SPINAL-EPIDURAL ANALGESIA (CSE)

In recent years some units have introduced the technique of CSE. Labour analgesia is provided by an intrathecal dose of opioid, local anaesthetic or a combination of both. An epidural catheter is placed at the same time as subarachnoid injection. Subarachnoid opioid blockade is rarely adequate for later stages of labour and epidural analgesia can then be introduced. When the technique is used it is usually part of an ambulatory analgesia policy. Advantages include very rapid onset of analgesia, reduced doses of local anaesthetic. Potential disadvantages include insertion of the epidural catheter into the subarachnoid space, drug flux from epidural to subarachnoid space, the potential for meningitis and difficulty interpreting epidural test doses. Post dural puncture headache is generally infrequent. The technique is effective and safe in experienced hands and is associated with very high levels of maternal satisfaction.

EFFECTS OF ANALGESIA ON PROGRESS AND OUTCOME OF LABOUR

Good quality analgesia is likely to enhance the progress of labour and increase cooperation by reducing maternal catacholamine levels, acidosis and exhaustion. Physical and psychological methods of analgesia and entonox have no demonstrable effect on labor progression. Opioids, particularly morphine, in large doses reverse the stimulatory effects of oxytocin on myometrical activity. Most interest in analgesia and labour progression focusses on regional analgesia. Poorly performed regional analgesia produces regional anaesthesia, motor weakness, inability to cooperate, and necessitates bed rest. Local anaesthetics can produce transient delays in uterine activity which are prolonged with very high doses. Well managed regional analgesia produces excellent analgesia, reduces maternal acidosis, retains power sensation of contractions and co-operation. Recumbency is not necessary and ambulation may be possible. The effect of regional analgesia on labour remains controversial, it may prolong the latent phase of labour and increase interventional delivery, particularly in primiparae. Outcome advantages of labour with ambulation have yet to be confirmed. Should interventional delivery be needed regional analgesia allows painless delivery without general anaesthesia.

ANALGESIA FOLLOWING OPERATIVE DELIVERY

Up to 20% of women deliver by caesarian section. Regional analgesic techniques established in labour or preoperatively will provide pain relief in the early postoperative period. The aims of subsequent analgesia are:

- to allow early mobilization of the mother
- to allow normal maternal interaction with the newborn
- negligible maternal side-effects
- negligible transfer of analgesics across placenta or into milk
- negligible fetal side-effects.

For a discussion of parenteral and oral drugs suitable in the postoperative period see Chapter 10.

SECTION 3

PAIN OF CANCER AND ADVANCED HIV DISEASE

CHAPTER 14

CANCER PAIN

It has been estimated by the WHO that every day four million people throughout the world are suffering from cancer pain, the prevalence of which rises with disease progression. At the time of diagnosis 50% of patients are suffering from pain; by the time the disease is advanced this proportion has risen to 80%. Cancer pain is still ineffectively treated, although there are well described guidelines for its management using simple and inexpensive pharmacological therapy. It has been demonstrated that 90% of patients can obtain good pain relief when these guidelines are followed.

In order to treat cancer pain effectively the clinician must have an idea of its likely pathophysiology, the clinical pharmacology of the most commonly used analgesic drugs, and other techniques which may be needed if these are not completely successful. In addition, the physician must have a wider understanding of pain so that the **person who has the pain** and his or her goals and values are at the centre of its management. Effective pain relief often involves teamwork: the patient and family form its heart and other members join and leave as the illness and the needs of the patient change. Cancer pain is a dynamic condition – because of disease progression, the changing psychological, social and spiritual state of the patient and the plasticity of the CNS – and therefore treatment needs to be constantly reviewed. Cancer pain needs active continuous therapy throughout the course of the disease.

DEFINITION OF TERMS USED IN CANCER PAIN

Pain is a somatopsychic experience, i.e. it is an experience that affects, and is affected by, both the mind and the body. It involves the perception of a painful stimulus by the nervous system (nociception) and the reaction of a person to this – pain is the personal experience of nociception. Pain is experienced by people; nociception describes what is understood to go on in pain receptors, neural pathways and in experimental preparations. Many influences modulate the neurophysiological signals to produce the individual's experience of pain. The **plasticity** of the nervous system is a key concept which has already been described (see Chapter 1). It is important to try and classify different types of pain, but also remember that this can lead to oversimplification of a complex experience.

Nociceptive pain

This is chronic pain for which there is an identifiable lesion causing tissue damage, accompanied by stimulation of nociceptors in somatic or visceral structures. The damage is outside the central or peripheral nervous system. Nociceptive pain can be further subdivided into somatic and visceral pain.

Somatic pain. In cancer pain somatic pain is related to tumour infiltration of somatic ('bodily') structures such as bone or muscle. It is commonly described by sufferers as having 'aching', 'stabbing' or 'throbbing' qualities.

Visceral pain. This is related to a lesion in, or tumour infiltration or compression of, a hollow viscus or solid organ with an autonomic innervation. It may be described in terms such as 'gnawing' or 'cramping' (for example the pain of partial bowel obstruction). It may be 'aching', 'sharp' or 'throbbing' when a solid organ, its capsule or a mesentery is involved.

In clinical practice nociceptive pain is likely to be responsive to opioids and other primary analgesics.

Neuropathic pain

Neuropathic pain results from and is sustained by nerve damage, in either the central or the peripheral nervous system. It is suggested by abnormal sensation or pain in a region of motor, sensory or autonomic dysfunction. These abnormal sensations may be very subtle and are easily missed. Patients may describe the pain as having a 'burning', 'tingling' or 'numbing' quality. Sometimes patients suffer intolerable itching. Clinicians often use the term **lancinating** for the intermittent 'electric shock-like' shooting pain that patients may describe when there is nerve damage.

Neuropathic pains may be only poorly responsive to opioids or, arguably, not responsive to them at all. Secondary analgesics or more specialized pain therapy may be needed and only partial relief ever achieved. A fuller discussion of this subject is found in Chapter 19.

Referred pain

Pain may be felt in a superficial or deep structure some distance from its anatomical source. There are different types of referred pain – the mechanisms of some are at least partially understood (e.g. the pain that accompanies nerve damage in spinal cord compression), but others are more complex. Examples commonly seen in clinical practice include back pain from carcinoma of the pancreas and shoulder pain of hepatic origin.

Idiopathic pain

This term is controversial, as it is used when pain is said to be disproportionate to the known disease that is present. **Pain, whatever its aetiology, is as bad as the patient says it is**. Pain can predate, or never be associated with, physical signs and a structural lesion is not always shown by even the most sophisticated imaging equipment. Medical, and where necessary surgical, treatments must be used appropriately before labelling pain idiopathic. A psychological awareness should always guide the care of a person suffering pain, whatever the cause. Specialist psychological and psychiatric treatments are sometimes required for pain therapy. Complementary therapies too may be helpful, and research is in progress to try and define for whom they are most useful. It may be more fruitful to consider idiopathic pain as 'opioid-irrelevant pain.'

Opioid-irrelevant pain

Dr John Hinton, a psychiatrist, used this term to describe those cancer pains, or aspects of pain, which are not amenable to pharmacological or other medical therapy. Pain that presents physically may be the expression of personal and family torment which, if not addressed, is likely to lead to unrelieved pain. Many patients with the most difficult pains have the elements of **spiritual, psychological, social and physical pain** mixed together. The patient's anguish may itself cause **staff pain** – distress and division within the multi disciplinary team of people caring for the patient. The source of this division must be recognized and great efforts made to keep the team communicating and together in order to contain the anguish of the patient and their family. Dame Cicely Saunders has called pain with all these elements '**total pain**'.

For diagnostic and therapeutic purposes cancer pain has been divided into three main categories:

- Pain from the tumour itself, at primary and/or secondary sites
- Pain arising from treatment of the tumour
- Pain due to a concurrent non-malignant cause or pre-existing illness: guidance on management will be found under the appropriate section elsewhere in this book.

PAIN FROM THE TUMOUR ITSELF

Pain which can be said to arise directly from the effects of the tumour can itself be subdivided according to its temporal pattern:

- **Acute pain** – from a pathological fracture, for example
- **Chronic pain** – this is difficult to define in cancer pain: any pain that needs continuing analgesia to contain it is chronic. Whereas patients with chronic non-malignant pain can wait some time before assessment in a pain clinic, patients with cancer pain need to be seen urgently. The pain experience is different.
- **Incident pain** – is absent at rest but brought on by a particular manoeuvre, for example coughing, walking or turning. The manoeuvre may be voluntary or involuntary.
- **Breakthrough pain** – defined as 'intermittent exacerbations of a pain otherwise well controlled with appropriate doses of analgesia': it can encompass incident pain. Some breakthrough pains are very short-lived but extremely severe. They may be somatic, visceral or neuropathic in aetiology.

ASSESSING THE PATIENT WITH CANCER PAIN: THE FIRST INTERVIEW

Unless the patient is in severe pain the first interview should have broader aims than simply assessing the pain and starting to treat it. Some other important ones are outlined below.

Gaining the patient's confidence

It is important to gain both the patient's and the family's confidence. You will need time to read the referral letter and notes beforehand, as these are often very lengthy for people with cancer. Patients will often be accompanied by a friend or family member who they may want to be present for the interview. Make sure that you speak to the patient and the companion separately at some point, with the patient's agreement. Sit down with the patient with as much privacy as possible (such interviews sometimes take place on a busy ward). Discourage outside interruptions and make it clear that you have made time solely for the purpose of listening to that patient and finding out his or her concerns. Past bereavements are often very near the surface: acknowledge these and any other problems that are mentioned, even if they are not central to the present interview, before moving on. You may not be able to do anything about them but reacting shows that you have heard and that the patient's feelings and emotions are important to you. This may be therapeutic in itself.

Finding out the patient's priorities

Cancer is a multisystem disorder and the patient may have a wide range of symptoms: some may be more important to the patient than pain. These problems may not be completely 'soluble', or you may need to refer to another medical specialist or professional for appropriate help. Remember that analgesic drugs have adverse effects which may exacerbate pre-existing complications of cancer or its treatment: for example, if a patient is already troubled by nausea it will be necessary to try and control this and prevent further opioid-induced emesis. All the patient's present difficulties, medical and non-medical, will affect pain control.

Patient's insight

One of the most taxing components of the initial interview can be finding out what the patient knows about his or her illness. Patients undergoing radical treatment regimens with the aim of cure are usually fully informed about their illness, but do not assume this. Patients with advanced disease may be fully aware of what is happening but may be using a number of psychological defences, including denial, to cope. It is not necessary to confront this and make the patient 'face' their impending death. Many patients die without seeming to acknowledge what is happening. It *is* necessary to find out if the patient has all the information he or she wants and whether their psychological strategy is effective in keeping the inevitable fear and anxiety within manageable limits for most of the time. The ability to communicate effectively and compassionately with patients, carers and colleagues is a vital skill in pain management.

Is the patient depressed?

It is not inevitable for a patient with cancer to be depressed. It is normal for patients to go through stages of feeling low and needing extra support when they are adjusting to new circumstances (the time of diagnosis, the finding of metastatic disease etc.). This is often called an 'adjustment reaction'. Depression is both underdiagnosed and undertreated in cancer patients. Many of the somatic symptoms of depression are common in cancer itself (anorexia, weight loss, alterations in sleep pattern). It is useful to ask about **anhedonia** – the inability to take pleasure in anything. Even patients with advanced disease will get pleasure from seeing friends, for example. If there is nothing that gives someone's life joy and meaning then depression is a possible cause. Other important symptoms of depression unrelated to the physical illness include feelings of guilt and worthlessness.

A pain history

In order to treat cancer pain effectively the clinician must attempt to diagnose the cause of each pain the patient has.

> **About 86% of patients with cancer have more than one pain and 34% of patients have four or more pains. As many as half of these are not caused by the cancer itself. Take a careful history and make a plan of management for each pain. Start with the worst one.**

The pain history is discussed fully in Chapter 9. In the patient with cancer pain the clinician must pay particular attention to the following features:

- **Pain present at rest** – back pain, persisting when the patient is at rest, may be the first sign of spinal cord compression. This is fully discussed in Chapter 16.
- **Incident pain** – a full history of precipitating manoeuvres is needed for assessment and management.
- **Response to analgesics** – many patients will have already tried analgesics, either bought over the counter or prescribed by another clinician. Careful questioning is necessary to find out exactly which medicines have been of help, what doses have been tried and what adverse effects have occurred.

- **The quality of sleep** – anxiety, pain and depression may all disrupt sleep and lower the patient's pain threshold. A frequent early goal in pain management is for the patient to have a good night's sleep.
- **Identifying difficult pains** – with experience it will be possible to identify those pains that may be difficult to relieve completely or which may need more than primary analgesics. These include incident pain, neuropathic pain and 'total pain'.
- **The patient's interpretation of what is causing the pain** – this will often give an indication of the patient's insight into the cancer or his or her concerns about treatment. It may also reveal misconceptions or misunderstandings that need further discussion.

> **Remember**: a full medical, psychosocial and family history is needed to manage cancer pain.

It may not be appropriate to complete the pain history at a first meeting and different members of the team may collect different parts of the story.

- A **family history** may reveal that the patient has watched a relative die in unrelieved pain from cancer, which will affect his or her expectations of the current illness. This may only be discovered on direct questioning.
- The **psychosocial history** will reveal not only non-medical pressures that may exacerbate pain, but also the family and friends around who may be able to offer the patient support of various kinds.

Physical examination

Do not neglect this, even in a patient who has been seen by many other doctors. If there is reason to curtail it at the first meeting it should be completed at another time. New findings which may lead to either further antitumour or palliative treatment have been shown to follow from a comprehensive and repeated assessment of the pain patient, particularly one who has advanced disease.

Investigations

These must be appropriate to the individual. Many young patients receiving curative cancer treatment will already have been extensively investigated for staging of the tumour and monitoring treatment. An elderly patient with advanced cancer may be receiving palliation only, and more sophisticated investigations may be both uncomfortable and peripheral to the aims of treatment. For example, soft-tissue imaging, by MRI or CT scanning, may be the only investigation that can establish the cause of difficult neuropathic pains such as lumbosacral plexopathy, but it may not be appropriate for every individual. Using the information from the history and knowledge of the particular tumour may be the best guide for that person. Conversely, an investigation which demonstrates an 'untreatable' lesion may sometimes be a great help, both for pain management and to give prognostic information to the patient.

- **! Remember that although open scanners are becoming available, an MRI involves the patient lying flat in a narrow tunnel for up to half an hour. They will also hear loud banging noises.**
- **! Remember that a patient must be able to lie flat for at least 20 minutes to have a CT scan.**
- **Both will involve transport off the ward, and even to another hospital.**

CANCER PAIN SYNDROMES

BONE PAIN

Metastatic bone disease is the most common cause of pain in cancer patients, but not all bony deposits cause pain. It has been shown that 25% of patients with known secondary bone disease remain entirely pain free, and that some patients with documented, widespread disease feel pain at only a few sites.

The quality of pain from bony metastases varies from a dull aching to an experience of overwhelming severity which is intensified by specific movements, or on weight bearing if the long bones are affected. This is a type of incident pain.

Pathophysiology

Bony deposits cause pain by several mechanisms, including:

- stretching or distortion of the periosteum/endosteum, activating nociceptors
- tumour growth into surrounding soft tissues
- tumour infiltration/compression of adjacent nerves by tumour growth or bony collapse
- tumour growth causing weakening of the bone and eventual collapse
- chemical pain mediators being released from the bone and activating nociceptors
- reactive muscle spasm
- microfractures and pathological fractures.

Management of bone pain

This is treated by three main modalities:

- **Primary analgesics** – using the WHO Analgesic Ladder (see Chapter 2).
- **Radiotherapy** – this is the treatment of choice when there is localized metastatic bone pain. The dose is usually given as a single fraction and adverse effects are unusual. Hemi-body irradiation could be used for widespread pain (for example in carcinoma of the prostate), but the likelihood of toxicity is greater. Intravenous radioactive strontium-89 can also be given for more generalized pain but it is expensive and its exact indications have not been fully established.
- **Treatment of the underlying disease** by specific hormonal or cytotoxic chemotherapy such as tamoxifen for a postmenopausal patient with breast cancer.

Bisphosphonates in the treatment of pain from metastatic bone disease

Bisphosphonates are finding a place in the control of bony pain as well as the prevention of skeletal complications in patients with metastatic bone disease and multiple myeloma. Current evidence for an analgesic effect is best for pamidronate disodium. This is given as an infusion over 2 hours, at doses of 60–90 mg every 2–4 months for as long as necessary, and has been shown to reduce both the incidence of bone pain and skeletal complications. It is not yet a first-line treatment for bone pain.

Pathological fracture

Large lytic metastatic lesions in long bones will predispose a patient to a 'pathological fracture', i.e. a fracture that occurs with minimal or no trauma to the bone (see below).

BACK PAIN IN CANCER PATIENTS

The vertebral column is the most common site for bony metastases (the commonest primary tumours being lung, breast and prostate cancers) and there are a number of specific vertebral column syndromes, which are listed in Table 14.1. It is essential to make an accurate, early diagnosis of the cause of back pain in the cancer patient because epidural extension of the tumour causing spinal cord or cauda equina compression is the second most common neurological complication of cancer. **It is an oncological emergency**. Of patients with spinal cord compression 90% report back pain at some point. Treatment needs to be instituted before neurological sequelae are present, as these are not usually reversible and a patient may be left with disastrous paraplegia and double incontinence for the rest of a considerably shortened life.

Spinal cord compression

Spinal cord compression may be the first manifestation of malignancy – the most common cause is posterior extension of the tumour from the vertebral body into the epidural space. More rarely the tumour can:

- extend from the posterior arch of a vertebra
- infiltrate through the intervertebral foramen into the epidural space from the paravertebral region.

> **The thoracic spine is involved in 70% of patients with spinal cord compression, 20% for the lumbosacral region and 10–15% for the cervical region. Have a high index of suspicion in the cancer patient who complains of rest pain in the thoracic region, particularly if there is bony tenderness.**

History

The earliest symptom for most patients with spinal cord compression is **back pain**, and this may precede neurological complications by a considerable period. Back pain is very common both in the general population and in the cancer patient without spinal cord compression, so characteristic symptoms and signs must be actively sought. The patient may have a history of lung, breast or prostate cancer, or another tumour that is known to spread to bone.

Pain characteristics particularly associated with spinal cord compression:

- Rapidly progressive back pain in a crescendo pattern
- Radicular pain, which may be unilateral or bilateral
- Back/radicular pain exacerbated by sneezing, coughing and other sudden movements
- Back pain exacerbated by lying down and partially relieved on standing or sitting
- Back pain present at rest, especially if severe enough to interrupt sleep at night
- The patient may notice electric shock sensations extending down the length of the spine when the neck is flexed (Lhermitte's sign)

Neurological symptoms

As compression of the cord progresses patients will complain of leg weakness and difficulty in walking, climbing stairs etc. They will have progressive sensory loss below the level of the lesion and autonomic dysfunction will develop. At the beginning these symptoms may be very subtle and are often overlooked by patient and doctor alike. Slowly progressive weakness has a better prognosis for functional recovery after treatment than if this process is rapid. Bladder and bowel dysfunction will occur late in the course of the syndrome.

Signs on examination may include:

- **Bony tenderness on palpation** – often at a spinal level consistent with signs of neurological deficit
- **Loss of joint position/vibration sense** – epidural extension will frequently involve the dorsal columns first
- **A sensory level** – if compression is advanced, earlier presentation will be accompanied by altered pinprick sensation. Altered thermal sensation may sometimes precede this. Saddle anaesthesia may be present in cauda equina compression
- **Motor weakness, spastic or flaccid paralysis** – depending on the stage and rapidity of process
- **Reduced anal tone** on rectal examination and a full bladder if sphincter dysfunction is present
- **Lhermitte's sign** – i.e. sudden electric shocks present along the length of the spine on cervical flexion.

Investigation and treatment

The non-specialist should seek expert assessment and guidance immediately from a clinical oncologist and details of treatment will not be presented here. Investigation should include the whole spinal column, and an MRI with pre- and post-contrast enhancement is becoming the investigation of choice. Myelography is rarely used nowadays. Immediate treatment with high-dose corticosteroids (e.g. dexamethasone 16 mg p.o. daily and reducing thereafter) is appropriate in all but the very sickest patients. Other treatment modalities will be chosen depending on the patient's general condition, the tumour type, and the stage and grade of the disease. These include radiotherapy, neurosurgery and chemotherapy.

> **Early diagnosis and appropriate treatment are vital in preventing distressing irreversible neurological morbidity in cancer patients. A delay of hours in seeking appropriate advice and treatment could be disastrous. Spine radiographs can be normal in patients with epidural tumour.**

Other causes of back pain in cancer patients

Back pain may have a non-malignant origin in the cancer patient but an expert oncological opinion is needed for appropriate management when there is the possibility of primary or secondary disease in the vertebral column.

TABLE 14.1 Cancer pain syndromes associated with direct tumour involvement of vertebral bodies

Vertebral body syndromes	*Symptoms and signs*
Odontoid process syndrome C1 involvement may result in pathological fracture, subluxation, and spinal cord or brainstem compression. Usually associated with invasion of the atlas. Note: MRI most useful investigation	Severe neck pain radiating over posterior aspect of the skull and vertex. Pain exacerbated by neck movement, especially flexion. Progressive sensory and motor signs begin in upper extremities; spinal cord compression may be insidious. Pain localized to adjacent paraspinal area
C7–T1 syndrome Tumour spread may be haematogenous, or along nerves from tumour originating in brachial plexus or paravertebral space to adjacent vertebral body and epidural space. Note: CT/MRI of cervical and thoracic regions necessary in patients with interscapular pain	Constant dull ache, radiating to both shoulders and interscapular region. Tenderness on percussion over spinous processes at this level. Radicular pain, usually unilateral, in posterior arm, elbow and ulnar aspect of hand. Horner's syndrome may be present
T12–L1 syndrome Note: imaging of pelvic bones alone will miss cause of pain	Dull, aching, mid-back pain exacerbated by lying or sitting, relieved by standing. Pain can radiate in girdle-like band anteriorly or to both paraspinal and lumbosacral area. May be referred to sacroiliac joint and/or superior iliac crest
Sacral syndrome Most frequent in patients with gynaecological, genitourinary, colon or breast cancers	Destruction of sacrum leads to severe, aching, focal pain in low back or coccygeal area, radiating to buttocks, perineum or posterior thighs. Insidious onset. Exacerbated by lying, sitting; relieved by walking. Increasing pain with perianal sensory loss. Bowel, bladder dysfunction and impotence may develop. Lateral extension may cause incident pain in hip. Local invasion of sacral plexus may occur

BASE OF SKULL DISEASE

Tumours that metastasize to bone (most commonly lung, breast and prostate tumours) may cause symptoms and signs in the base of the skull (Table 14.2). The cranial nerves exit through the basal foramina and are often involved when secondary and, less frequently, primary cancers are present in this region. Plain radiographs are often normal and an MRI scan is the best investigation for localizing the tumour. Discuss the most useful investigation for an individual patient with the radiologist.

TABLE 14.2 Cancer pain syndromes associated with direct tumour involvement of the base of the skull

Named by area of direct tumour involvement	*Signs and symptoms*
Orbital syndrome Note: often diagnosed earlier than other base of skull syndromes because of proptosis	Increasing pain in retroorbital/supraorbital area of affected eye. Blurred vision/diplopia may occur. On examination proptosis, chemosis, ispilateral papilloedema, external ophthalmoparesis, decreased sensation in ophthalmic division of Vth nerve. Decreased visual acuity
Parasellar syndrome (cavernous sinus syndrome)	Unilateral headache (frontal, supraorbital), ocular paresis (diplopia) without proptosis. Papilloedema may be present, visual field defects on testing
Middle fossa (gasserian ganglion) **syndrome** Note: on examination patients may have weakness of ipsilateral muscles on mastication. Sensory symptoms in distribution of Vth cranial nerve may precede others by weeks/months	Facial numbness, paraesthesia and pain which is commonly referred to cheek/jaw (distribution of V_2 and V_3). Pain quality may be dull, continuous ache or paroxysmal and lancinating. Other neurological symptoms may be present but trigeminal sensory symptoms most common
Jugular foramen syndrome	Hoarseness and/or dysphagia and/or dysarthria. Occipital pain, referred to vertex of head, behind involved ear, ipsilateral shoulder or neck. Exacerbated by movement, local tenderness often present. Horner's syndrome, weakness of sternocleidomastoid and trapezius, ptosis may be present. Glossopharyngeal neuralgia (lancinating throat pain) may be present and is sometimes sole complaint
Clivus syndrome	Vertex headache exacerbated by neck flexion. Lower cranial nerve (VI–XII) dysfunction begins unilaterally, progresses to bilateral weakness (facial weakness, hoarseness, dysphagia, dysarthria, trapezius muscle weakness)
Sphenoid sinus syndrome	Severe bifrontal headache radiating to both temples. Intermittent retro-orbital pain. Nasal stuffiness, fullness in head, diplopia, unilateral or bilateral VIth nerve palsy may be present
Occipital condyle syndrome Note: XIIth nerve involvement possible	Severe, localized, continuous, unilateral occipital pain exacerbated by neck flexion

Treatment

This will involve:

- standard analgesic therapy following the WHO Analgesic Ladder guidelines
- irradiation of the metastatic cancer
- standard antitumour treatment (for primary or secondary disease).

> **Pain may precede neurological signs and symptoms by many weeks or months. Early diagnosis leads to more successful treatment.**

Pain can also result from the treatment of cancer: this can involve surgery, radiotherapy and chemotherapy.

Acute postoperative pain is described in Chapter 10, but some chronic syndromes are listed in Table 14.3.

PAIN SYNDROMES DUE TO RADIATION DAMAGE

Pathophysiology

Radiation tissue damage involves fibrosis, inflammation, soft tissue ischaemia and necrosis. A second primary neoplasm can arise in tissue irradiated many years previously and present with pain.

> **It is always important to distinguish postradiation pain from tumour recurrence: both tend to occur late in the course of the patient's illness.**

Treatment

Prevention of radiation syndromes by careful assessment of dose and delivery of radiotherapy is the most important component of pain management. Once established, the chronic syndromes that follow radiation damage can only be treated symptomatically, and when they involve nerve damage (neuropathic pain) this may be difficult (Table 14.4).

POST-CHEMOTHERAPY SYNDROMES

There is no general treatment for these as the causes are so variable. Standard pain therapy regimens should be followed and additional points are made in Table 14.5.

TABLE 14.3 Post-surgical pain syndromes

Syndrome	*Signs and symptoms*
Post-thoracotomy: caused by injury to intercostal nerves by surgical incision or retractors	Needs careful evaluation: pain which returns after original postoperative resolution (at 1–2 months) commonly due to tumour recurrence. Non-malignant intercostal nerve-damage pain is typically burning in quality, associated with dysaesthesias and intermittent stabbing pain in scar area and surrounding hyperpathia. Pain worse with movement, and frozen shoulder may develop. Resolves with time. Investigate (CT) persisting/worsening pain
Postmastectomy: caused by interruption of intercostobrachial nerve (T1–3), usually by axillary dissection. Anatomically very wide range of size and distribution of nerve, and hence variation in distribution/severity of pain	Reported in 4–10% of women undergoing breast surgery. Pain in posterior/medial aspects of arm, axilla and anterior chest wall. Pain may start immediately or as long as 18 months after surgery (look for chest wall recurrence if starts after this). Pain described as tight, constricting, with burning quality. Exacerbated by movement, which may lead to frozen shoulder. O/E sensory change in painful area. No associated lymphoedema
Post radical neck dissection: surgical damage to cervical plexus	Constant burning sensation in area of sensory loss. May be dysaesthesia and intermittent lancinating pain (unpleasant tingling and stinging)
Phantom limb syndromes: following amputation for cancer	1. Pain perceived to come from a limb that has been amputated 2. Pain in the stump of a limb that has been amputated

There are many postsurgical pain syndromes: not all are listed here. Scar pain may follow any operation. In cancer patients it is always important to be sure that pain is not due to tumour recurrence.

OTHER CANCER PAIN SYNDROMES

There are many pains associated with cancer that have not been specifically mentioned in this chapter, as their management follows the principles applicable to the general population. Some cancer pain syndromes with specific therapies are outlined below, but these should be used in addition to following the general rules of cancer pain management (regular oral medication using the WHO Pain Ladder etc.).

TABLE 14.4 Post-radiotherapy pain syndromes

Syndrome	*Symptoms and signs*
Radiation fibrosis of brachial plexus – may occur 6 months to 20 years after RT. Secondary to RT to upper chest/mediastinum for treatment of breast, lung cancer and lymphoma. More likely with higher doses of RT **NB**: upper plexus most commonly affected; if signs lower plexus be very wary of tumour infiltration. MRI/CT/EMG most important investigations	Pain uncommon. Predominant symptoms are numbness/paresthesiae and weakness in C5–6 distribution. (Thumb and index finger numbness, deltoid and biceps weakness.) Radiation skin changes and lymphoedema commonly associated Usually progressive, resulting in lymphoedematous, painful, useless arm
Radiation myelopathy – from irradiation of spinal cord. Uncommon **Risk**: irradiation for spinal cord compression or mediastinal therapy for oesophageal cancer/lymphoma. CT/MRI may be needed to exclude tumour recurrence.	Most often, burning dysaesthetic pain below level of irradiation precedes sensory, motor and autonomic changes. Usually within 1–2 years of RT but has been reported many years later. Sphincter involvement, weakness and spasticity occur later: usually progressive
Chronic radiation proctitis/enteritis **Risk**: pelvic and abdominal RT	Latency variable – months to years after RT. **Proctitis**: cramping abdominal pain, bloody diarrhoea and tenesmus. Strictures may cause partial bowel obstruction, fistulae may form. **Enteritis**: colicky abdominal pain +/– malabsorption
Osteoradionecrosis	Due to ischaemic tissue damage following radiotherapy. Leads to focal pain in area irradiated, sometimes many years after RT but more usually within 6 months

CARCINOMA OF THE PANCREAS

Various patterns of pain are recognized in this condition, depending on the site of the tumour, the pathways of local spread and the presence of distant metastases. This tumour is commonly advanced at the time of diagnosis.

Symptoms

Typically the pain is continuous, unvarying, midepigastric boring pain radiating through to the upper lumbar and lower thoracic region of the back. It is relieved by curling up and exacerbated by lying flat. Sometimes patients only have back pain. It is progressively severe.

The pain is often a mixture of somatic and visceral, and there may be neuropathic pain related to coeliac plexus invasion.

TABLE 14.5 Post-chemotherapy pain syndromes

Syndrome	*Symptoms and signs*
Oral mucositis – Most common with aggressive chemotherapy, e.g. in bone marrow transplant patients. Careful oral hygiene vital. **Note**: proctitis/colitis can also occur after high-dose radiotherapy to pelvis	Starts with intolerance to certain foods, progressing to erythema then muscosal ulceration and sloughing. Frequently extends to oesophagus and secondary fungal infection occurs. In most severe cases TPN needed temporarily. Usually peaks after 2–3 weeks. Treatment with local anaesthetic/antiseptic mouthwashes and opioids (PCA).
Symmetrical peripheral polyneuropathy – associated with treatment with vincristine (motor and sensory) or cis-platinum (mostly sensory)	Severe painful dysaesthesiae localized to feet and hands +/– allodynia. Acute jaw pain/claudication with vincristine. Resolves with reduction/end of chemotherapy. Treat as for neuropathic pain.
Steroid pseudorheumatism – associated with steroid dose reduction/withdrawal	Diffuse myalgias and arthralgias with muscle and joint tenderness. No signs joint inflammation. Fatigue and neuropsychological disturbances may occur. Treat by temporarily increasing steroid dose and withdrawing again at a slower rate
Aseptic necrosis of the femoral (humeral, less often) **head**. Complication of steroid therapy, can occur after only a few weeks. MRI investigation of choice	Hip or shoulder pain predates radiological signs by weeks/months. Reduction in range of joint movements. Pain relieved by rest. Use primary analgesics, occasionally joint replacement appropriate
Osteoporosis leading to crush fractures secondary to steroid therapy.	Attempts to prevent this with bisphosphonates being evaluated. Use lowest possible dose of steroids, for shortest possible time
Postherpetic neuralgia. Herpes zoster infection more common in cancer patients (immunosuppression and increasing age risk factors) and rash commonly occurs over the site of tumour or previous radiotherapy	Severe continuous burning pain in area of sensory loss, lancinating pains and painful dysaesthesiae all possible in different combinations

Pain therapy

Pharmacological therapy is often only partially successful and this pain often responds for a time to coeliac plexus block. A rare but catastrophic adverse effect of this procedure is paraplegia, which has made it unpopular in some centres.

INTRACRANIAL NEOPLASM

This may be primary or secondary cancer.

Symptoms

Raised intracranial pressure (ICP) and headache are not invariable, but typical features would be:

- headache worse in the morning or after lying flat
- headache exacerbated by coughing, straining at stool etc.
- associated with vomiting, but nausea less common.

Pain therapy

Steroid therapy to lower ICP often relieves headache, and a regular non-opioid may be as helpful as an opioid in relieving any residual pain.

PARTIAL BOWEL OBSTRUCTION

Abdominal and pelvic tumours of all types are associated with partial bowel obstruction but it is a particular risk with ovarian cancer, which frequently causes multiple peritoneal seedlings. The course is often one of relapses and remissions for both obstruction and abdominal pain. The bowel symptoms may arise both from physical narrowing of the bowel lumen by invasion and compression by tumour masses and nerve plexus involvement, causing bowel dysfunction.

Symptoms

- Colicky abdominal pain, often against a background of constant visceral pain
- Colic may be relieved by the patient holding a heating pad over or applying pressure to the painful area.

Pain is often associated with:

- constipation and/or diarrhoea
- vomiting, which may be infrequent but copious
- nausea.

Pain therapy

Surgery

Expert assessment is needed before surgery is undertaken as it is often both inappropriate and ineffective in patients with advanced disease.

Medical management
Opioids and antispasmodics (e.g. hyoscine butylbromide) are needed for pain therapy. They may be administered subcutaneously in patients unable to tolerate oral medication. Prokinetic drugs may exacerbate pain and other symptoms. Faecal softeners and antiemetics are also used.

HEPATIC PAIN

Tumour infiltration of the liver can cause painful stretching of the liver capsule, though this is not invariably present with liver metastases.

Symptoms
A dull aching pain in the right subcostal region is common and it may radiate to the right shoulder. Hepatic pain may also present with symptoms in the right mid and lower back. Superimposed acute pain may develop, possibly due to haemorrhage into a metastasis: this will usually resolve over the course of a week, but extra medication will be needed over this period.

The pain may be associated with:

- anorexia
- nausea
- postprandial vomiting/epigastric pain occur when there is massive hepatomegaly ('squashed stomach').

N.B: Pain in this region may also be due to gallbladder distension with biliary obstruction.

PELVIC PAIN

This may accompany colorectal and female reproductive tract tumours. It is also associated with primary tumours affecting the pelvic bones and those of the distal genitourinary tract.

Symptoms
Constant aching pain (rectal or perineal) which is often exacerbated by sitting or walking about. Patients may have to lie on their side or sit on a rubber ring to be comfortable.

Pain therapy
This pain is often difficult to control and secondary analgesics, adjuvant drugs or special techniques may be required.

TENESMOID PAIN

This accompanies rectal tumour recurrence and other pelvic tumours involving the presacral plexus.

Symptoms

A painful sensation of rectal fullness accompanied by a dull aching pain. Patients often complain of an intermittent, severe stabbing pain shooting up through the rectum.

Pain therapy

This is often a difficult pain and secondary analgesics, adjuvant drugs and special techniques may be required.

CONSTIPATION

Constipation may be severe enough to cause significant abdominal pain. Patients with advanced cancer may have a number of risk factors:

- constipating drugs such as opioids and drugs with anticholinergic effects, e.g. tricyclics
- paraplegia (spinal cord compression)
- immobility
- dehydration and poor diet.

Symptoms

These may mimic those of partial bowel obstruction, with colicky abdominal pain and other GI symptoms.

Detection

Prevention of constipation in this high-risk group of patients is vital. History and examination are important (faeces will be palpable on abdominal examination). A plain abdominal film will confirm faecal loading.

Pain therapy includes:

- standard pharmacological approach
- active treatment of the underlying condition, with prevention of further episodes using oral and rectal measures as necessary.

MYOFASCIAL PAIN

This is discussed more fully in Chapter 17. Myofascial pain is not uncommon but is certainly underdiagnosed in cancer patients. Pain is related to hypersensitive trigger point(s) and the patient 'jumps' when touched there. Injection of these trigger points with local anaesthetic may help.

ACUTE PAIN

Many of the acute pain syndromes are common to the general population (e.g. postoperative pain) and should receive similar treatment. A special problem for cancer patients is that much acute pain is acute-on-chronic and many are taking long-term morphine therapy; often such patients are undertreated when they are prescribed analgesia for the new pain.

If a patient with advanced cancer is receiving opioids for chronic pain ensure that the increase in opioid dose gives adequate analgesia for any acute event. The dose may seem very high to someone unused to using opioids for cancer pain: do not hesitate to contact a palliative care or pain physician for guidance or reassurance.

PATHOLOGICAL FRACTURE

This is a fracture which occurs after minimal or no trauma. Both incipient and completed fractures are an important cause of incident pain and acute pain in cancer patients.

Risk factors are tumours that metastasize to bone, e.g. breast, lung, prostate, renal cell and thyroid.

Symptoms

Pain on weight-bearing, progressing to pain at rest.

Detection

Radiographic findings which suggest a high risk of pathological fracture include:

- a large lytic lesion in the peritrochanteric region
- any lesion involving two-thirds of the bony cortex.

NB: Both lytic and sclerotic metastases represent areas of bone weakened by tumour.

Pain therapy

Where appropriate for the patient, **internal fixation** is the treatment of choice as it relieves pain, increases mobility and prevents the protracted, damaging bed-rest associated with conservative management.

Other modalities include:

- analgesia
- radiotherapy
- systemic antitumour treatment.

When a patient sustains a fracture and internal fixation is either impossible or inappropriate he or she should be nursed in a suitable bed (e.g. 'air-loss') so that movement of the fracture site, and therefore pain, is minimized. Intraspinal pain therapy may be necessary.

CYTOTOXIC DRUG ADMINISTRATION

Many drugs used in the treatment of cancer can cause tissue damage if extravasated. Examples include daunorubicin and vincristine. There are several types of pain associated with cytotoxic drug administration including:

- venous spasm – pain occurs along the line of the vein into which the drug is being administered. It is reduced by slowing the infusion rate
- chemical phlebitis – pain and erythema develop as the drug is infused, and the vein may become thrombosed
- drug extravasation – this can cause such extensive tissue damage that plastic surgery is required. Each unit will have a protocol to be followed in this event, but pharmacological pain therapy should not be forgotten.

STARTING PAIN THERAPY IN THE CANCER PATIENT

To delay treatment until the definitive cause of a cancer pain has been defined is unnecessary: for the great majority of cancer patients pharmacological therapy, coupled with appropriate antitumour treatment, will be the mainstay of management.

> **Whatever treatment is started it must be kept under constant review. Cancer pain is a dynamic condition that changes with changes in the patient's disease and psychological and social state.**

When starting a pain therapy be certain to spend some time explaining:

- the possible adverse effects of treatment
- how long the treatment will need to be tried before any improvement can be expected
- other possible treatment options if the first is unsuccessful
- the degree of pain relief that you expect to be able to obtain for each pain the patient has
- that you need feedback from the patient about adverse drug effects and the success or otherwise of your pain therapies in order to give the best possible management.

Initial treatment

Whatever stage the patient's cancer has reached, opioids of appropriate strength and/or NSAIDs (primary analgesics) should be prescribed and **used regularly**. Antitumour treatment may take time both to organize and to take effect. Oral drug administration will be the best option for the great majority. For a few this will be impractical or contraindicated, and for an even smaller number with acute severe pain parenteral analgesia may be the only option to achieve rapid pain relief (see later, Practical guide to opioid therapy).

Using the WHO analgesic ladder (see Fig 2.1, p. 18)

When the patient is first seen:

- If the pain is mild, start a step 1 analgesic such as paracetamol or an NSAID.
- If the pain is moderate start a step 2 analgesic. These are weak opioids, most often in combination with a non-opioid, e.g. co-proxamol.
- If the patient is in severe pain start a step 3 analgesic such as morphine.

At every stage:

- move up the ladder if the pain is poorly controlled or the intensity increases; do not try another drug from the same step
- it is often worth continuing the non-opioid when a step 2 or 3 drug is introduced. Do not use two paracetamol-containing drugs at the same time
- use analgesics for cancer pain regularly, with 'rescue' doses for breakthrough pain available 'as required' (PRN).

> **The dose of analgesia can go down as well as up even in patients with advanced disease, particularly when another pain treatment therapy is being added (e.g. a nerve block). Titrate the dose against the pain.**

Treatment of the underlying tumour with curative or palliative intent will be a priority. Hormonal therapy, chemotherapy and radiotherapy are all used for both disease treatment and pain relief. Guidance from a clinical oncologist or palliative care physician is vital. Cancer is many different diseases – for some, even when the patient is frail and the disease very advanced, palliative treatment that will both extend and enhance life may be possible. What to use and when it is appropriate will depend on the patient's wishes and general condition, and the type, stage and grade of the tumour. The rule of constant review for efficacy and tolerability will particularly apply to a treatment given to someone with advanced disease. Once a treatment (e.g. chemotherapy) is started it does not have to be continued if it brings no benefit and is causing discomfort.

Examples of antitumour treatment that may be used in pain relief are:

- hormonal therapy, e.g. goserelin for prostate cancer, tamoxifen for breast cancer
- radiotherapy, e.g. single fractions for localized bony disease
- chemotherapy, e.g. for small cell lung cancer and multiple myeloma.

ADJUVANT DRUGS

These are given:

- to counter the adverse effects of an analgesic drug, e.g. laxatives for opioid-induced constipation (see Practical Guide to Opioid Therapy)
- as co-analgesics: for example dexamethasone may be used to reduce oedema round a tumour, thereby contributing to analgesia
- as psychotropic medication, for example amitriptyline for the treatment of depression
- as analgesics in their own right, e.g. anticonvulsants or antidepressants in neuropathic pain. Such drugs are sometimes called secondary analgesics (see below, Neuropathic Pains in Cancer).

INTRASPINAL THERAPY

This is used when other methods of administering drugs have failed. It usually consists of an epidural infusion, put in under local anaesthetic, with drugs administered into a fine-bore catheter from a syringe driver as a continuous infusion. Patients are often given the option to 'boost' the administration for breakthrough pain a certain number of times a day. Its use will be recommended and instituted by a pain clinic physician. Drugs given by this route do reach the systemic circulation and can cause unwanted effects, although the incidence is much smaller than when they are given orally as lower doses are used. There are special hazards associated with intraspinal therapy (see Chapter 2) and this technique involves a greater use of equipment, specialist medical and nursing time and greater inconvenience for the patient and his or her family.

The patient will need admission either to a pain relief unit (PRU) or hospice/hospital ward and the epidural infusion will require in-patient supervision and adjustment, after insertion, for 2–5 days at least. However, where pain is unrelieved by other means it may provide an answer. Once working successfully it can remain in place for weeks or months, and it is no barrier to domiciliary care.

Drugs commonly used by the intraspinal route for cancer pain include:

- opioids – morphine and diamorphine
- local anaesthetics – a synergistic effect has been demonstrated when a local anaesthetic is infused with opioid (e.g. bupivacaine in low concentration).

- clonidine may improve the efficacy of opioid/local anaesthetic mixtures
- intraspinal ketamine and midazolam are under investigation but are little used.

> **Remember**: Most cancer patients given epidural opioids will have been taking oral opioids. The dangers of respiratory depression are minimal if the dose is titrated against the pain.

Intraspinal therapy is used in cancer pain for:

- patients who have opioid-responsive pain but who are troubled by adverse effects with the drugs given systemically. About one-tenth the oral dose of opioid is needed epidurally
- the relief of pain from pathological fractures when the patient is too frail to undergo internal fixation or where this is inappropriate (e.g. crush fracture of a vertebra)
- the treatment of other types of incident pain, e.g. rib fractures causing pain on coughing
- the treatment of neuropathic pain or pains with a neuropathic component which have not responded to simpler therapy, e.g. chest wall pain from mesothelioma
- it may be used for other intractable pains, for example the management of pressure sore pain in a terminally ill patient (even when the danger of infection is present).

LOCAL ANAESTHETIC NERVE BLOCKS AND NEUROLYTIC BLOCKS

Between 2 and 5% of patients with advanced cancer receiving hospice care have nerve blocks as part of cancer pain management. A successful nerve block will allow smaller doses of opioid and NSAIDs to be used. Regional anaesthesia or single nerve blocks may be useful in **localized** cancer pain. Reversible anaesthesia with local anaesthetic drugs (and possibly steroids) may be used to interrupt nerve transmission in sympathetic or somatic nerves innervating a particular part of the body. Destroying the nerve, for example using a neurolytic drug such as phenol, is rarely performed now. Neurodestructive procedures are only used in patients with a short life expectancy where other simpler techniques have failed, because they have many potentially serious disadvantages, some of which are listed below:

- Even with nerve destruction the analgesia is not permanent and the block may have to be repeated, with an increased likelihood of morbidity.

- Complications arising from destruction of other nerves are long-lasting and may be very serious, such as paraplegia from a 'saddle block'.
- In time new deafferentation pain may develop in the area innervated by the damaged nerve(s).

Some examples are:

- **neurolytic coeliac plexus block** for carcinoma of the head of the pancreas and for pain affecting the proximal small bowel, liver and gallbladder. 80–90% of patients obtain good analgesia which lasts for 2–4 weeks; partial analgesia may last beyond this period. The most serious possible complication is paraplegia, which occurs in 1% of patients
- **neurolytic subarachnoid 'saddle block'** for perineal pain. A possible complication is loss of bladder and bowel sphincter control, and the technique is now most favoured in those patients with a catheter and colostomy already. Useful analgesia for bilateral saddle pain is obtained for 60% of patients and typically lasts some 2–4 weeks. Complications, of all sorts, occur in about 10% of patients.

Reversible local anaesthetic blocks can be used for immediate analgesia in acute pain, such as a fractured shaft of femur, especially when a patient needs to be moved before immobilization of the fracture site has been achieved. Analgesia from local anaesthetic blocks often outlasts the duration of the local anaesthetic itself, and the procedure can be repeated with minimal morbidity. It may also be possible to insert a catheter and infuse local anaesthetic to maintain analgesia.

Nerve blocks, whether permanent or temporary, rarely give complete pain relief and supplementary oral analgesia is usually required.

When a nerve block is successful the opioid dose may need to be greatly reduced to avoid sedation and possible respiratory depression.

NEUROSURGICAL NEUROABLATIVE TECHNIQUES

These involve destruction of the nerve supply to a localized part of the body, surgically or by thermal damage, to reduce pain. In **cordotomy** the anterolateral spinothalamic tract is interrupted to produce contralateral loss of pain and temperature sensation. In **rhizotomy** the nerve roots are sectioned. They are both most useful for nociceptive pain. Dysaesthetic pain may develop in the denervated region some months after both procedures. These techniques have been almost completely superseded by simpler and less hazardous treatments.

TREATMENT OF DEPRESSION

Depression may play a causal role in cancer pain and certainly lowers the patient's pain threshold. It has been repeatedly demonstrated that it is underdiagnosed and inadequately treated in all patients with cancer, whether or not they have pain.

Treatment modalities include:

- increased psychological and social support for the patient and family
- guidance from a psychiatrist, preferably one with a particular interest in oncology
- pharmacological treatment
- specialized palliative care.

OTHER ASPECTS OF PAIN RELIEF

A complete approach to pain therapy in the cancer patient should include the use of physical therapies such as occupational therapy and physiotherapy, with an individual patient assessment to make the best use of aids to daily living, walking aids, home adaptation etc. Many simple measures, such as the immobilization of a fracture site, can lead to significant pain relief. Pay attention to the detail of pain relief for an individual.

POSSIBLE REASONS FOR INADEQUATE PAIN RELIEF IN CANCER PATIENTS

There are many reasons why pain control may be inadequate even after a full patient assessment and the initiation of therapy. Some are listed below.

Clinician-related factors

Uncertainty about the role of opioid therapy:

- Patients with early disease
- Patients with indolent metastatic disease
- Patients with treatment-related pain.

Undertreatment

- Lack of knowledge of opioid therapy
- Incomplete assessment of the patient
- Lack of attention to the **person with the pain**
- Lack of attention to psychological, social and spiritual dimensions of pain
- Overestimation of risk of adverse drug reactions or opioid addiction
- Failure to review the effectiveness of an analgesic regimen
- Failure to spend enough time on initial patient education
- Failure to anticipate and prevent analgesic adverse effects, with consequent patient mistrust of the drug

- Failure to refer to other specialists when appropriate
- Failure to consider non-malignant causes of pain.

Patient-related factors

Ineffectual pain reporting:

- Only focusing on tumour treatment
- Stoicism
- Desire to please and 'not be a complainer'
- Use of pain as a monitor of disease progress
- Need to feel able to cope without drugs or other forms of therapy and support
- Cancer pain developing in the patient with chronic non-malignant pain.

Drug therapy

- Fear of addiction, particularly to opioids
- Fear that if morphine is used too soon the doctor will not have stronger drugs available 'when the pain gets really bad'
- Inadequate understanding of how to use opioids and other analgesics effectively
- Exaggerated fear of possible adverse effects of opioids
- Running out of analgesic drugs.

PALLIATIVE CARE

This has been defined by the WHO as the 'active total care of patients whose disease is not responsive to curative treatment'. Many patients with solid tumours (e.g. breast cancer) cannot be cured but much can be done to control the impact of the disease on the person and her or his family, and the patient may live with the disease for some years. Patients with the best oncological and palliative care still suffer immensely in ways that can never be fully alleviated (grief and loss, disfigurement and physical limitation from the illness etc.), but if this can be minimized by meticulous individual management then the patient is freer to choose how to spend his or her remaining time most fruitfully, within the limitations imposed by the illness.

Palliative care is not terminal care: many patients remain under the care of a hospice and its community team for some years, and in that time will be referred to other specialists for interventions to contain or alleviate the complications of cancer. Increasingly, patients with non-malignant pain are cared for by hospice teams in conjunction with other specialists. Palliative care is underpinned by:

- the concept that the psychological, spiritual and social care of the patient and his or her family is as important as the best medical care, and facilitated by it

- care of the individual: the patient's goals and needs are at the centre of good palliative care. Attention to detail and constant review of the objectives of therapy as the disease progresses are necessary to bring this about
- care of the family is an inextricable part of palliative care
- effective teamwork: the palliative care team will always comprise doctors and nurses (hospital and community), but other key professions include social workers, occupational and physiotherapists, chaplains (of all faiths) and bereavement counsellors. Other members of the team may include complementary therapists and volunteers. The palliative care team must work well with other professionals (oncologists, pain clinic physicians, family doctors, surgeons etc.) caring for the patient.

Role of the hospice and/or palliative care team in pain management

Patients with the most difficult types of cancer pain may be helped by referral for palliative care so that the physical, social, psychological and spiritual aspects of the pain may be intensively managed.

Total pain, neuropathic pain and incident pain may be very difficult to relieve even with expert help, but it is usually possible to make significant improvements in the quality of life of these patients and their families, and to support the staff caring for them.

TOTAL PAIN

This term was first used by Dame Cicely Saunders to describe patients experiencing intense suffering physically, spiritually, socially and psychologically. Most patients have some elements of all these aspects of pain, but not all feel them beyond endurance. Patients with total pain often do not have soluble problems, and a large measure of 'treatment' is containing the pain within limits acceptable for the patient, the family and the staff. Effective teamwork involving a specialized palliative care unit is a central part of management.

Suspect 'total pain' in:

- anyone who seems always to develop another physical symptom when one has been dealt with effectively: unless all the possible elements in their pain are addressed their distress may become unmanageable
- any dying young patient, particularly those with young families
- those who have been labelled 'difficult patients'
- those who have had a troubled life before the onset of the illness.

Be prepared to use specialized psychiatric and psychological help for these families.

NEUROPATHIC PAIN

This is considered in detail in Chapter 19. Neuropathic pain is a common element in cancer pain (see Table 14.6 for cancer pain syndromes with nerve involvement). Symptoms and signs of this condition should be sought and dealt with actively. Useful techniques include the following:

- Opioids in increasing doses until there is no longer a useful effect or the adverse effects become intolerable for the patient. If one fails an alternative strong opioid may then be tried.
- An antidepressant or an anticonvulsant may be added at this point, or used in conjunction with opioids from the beginning. There is no evidence to show that an antidepressant is superior to an anticonvulsant or vice versa. Analgesic effects start within 2–3 days and may go on increasing for 4–6 weeks. An anticonvulsant and antidepressant are then sometimes prescribed together.
- If these strategies are unhelpful then an epidural infusion containing opioid and a low concentration of bupivacaine may be used. Clonidine is sometimes added.
- A class 1 antidysrhythmic agent, a 'membrane stabilizing agent', such as mexilitene, can be tried.
- A subcutaneous ketamine infusion with or without an opioid may be used.
- If nerve compression by tumour is suspected then a trial of corticosteroids, in addition to other pain therapy, to reduce tumour oedema and so relieve pressure on the nerve is indicated. Try 4–8 mg dexamethasone o.d. for 5 days; if there is no improvement in this time, reduce and stop the steroid. If it has helped, reduce it gradually to the lowest effective dose.

TABLE 14.6 Cancer pain syndromes involving direct tumour involvement of nerve

Direct tumour involvement	*Symptoms and signs*
Epidural spinal cord and cauda equina compression. Symptoms vary with site of disease, multiple sites possible Oncological emergency MRI investigation of choice	>90% patients have back/neck pain as earliest symptom (local and/or radicular). Motor weakness leading to paraplegia. Sensory loss with level usually within 1 or 2 vertebral bodies of site of lesion. Loss of bowel and bladder function, late
Tumour-related mononeuropathy usually from tumour involving adjacent bony structure. Example: rib metastases – intercostal nerve	Constant burning pain in distribution of nerve. Hypoaesthesia and dysaesthesia in area of sensory loss is an early symptom
Paraneoplastic painful neuropathy	Both constant and paroxysmal dysaesthesia may predate symptoms and signs of some tumours (typically small-cell cancer lung). Sensory loss in extremities may be present.

TABLE 14.6 *(cont'd)*

Cervical plexopathy – anterior primary rami of C1–4 Infiltration/compression common in head and neck cancer or from metastases in cervical lymph nodes. Evaluate with CT/MRI	Pain in pre- and postauricular regions, anterior part of the neck. Pain may be referred to lateral aspects of face, neck and ipsilateral shoulder. Pain aching, burning or lancinating and exacerbated by neck movements or swallowing.
Brachial plexopathy – Associated with cancer of lung (Pancoast), breast, and, lymphoma from tumour enlarging adjacent lymph nodes or extension from lung. **Note:** CT/MRI scanning essential for accurate diagnosis Epidural extension very common	Pain almost universal and may predate neurological signs and symptoms by months. Lower plexus involvement (C8–T1): most common, pain radiates to elbow, medial forearm, ring and little fingers. Upper plexus (C5–6): pain in shoulder girdle, lateral arm and hand. Many patients progress to panplexopathy. Paraesthesias progress to weakness/numbness.
Lumbosacral plexopathy Associated with local extension of gynaecological, GU, colorectal cancers and sarcomas and lymphomas causing infiltration/compression Lumbar plexus: L1–4: (anterior primary rami) lies on paravertebral psoas muscle. Sacral plexus = L4–5 trunk and S1–3 (anterior primary rami)	Pain earliest symptom, dull, aching, constant. Upper plexopathy (30% patients): pain in back, lower abdomen, flank, iliac crest, anterolateral thigh. Sensory symptoms/signs in L1–4 distribution. May also have painful flexion of ipsilateral hip ('malignant psoas syndrome'). Lower plexopathy: most common, >50% patients. Usually pelvic tumour. Pain in buttocks, perineum, posterolateral part of leg. May have sensory changes/weakness in L5–S1 distribution. Bladder, bowel dysfunction, leg oedema may be present.
Sacral plexopathy – Occurs most frequently in patients with colon, genitourinary and gynaecological cancers. **Note:** CT/MRI scanning necessary to assess lumbosacral plexopathy	Dull, aching, midline pain. Local extension of a sacral/presacral mass. Sensory loss beginning in perianal area. Sensory findings are at first unilateral. Progression to bilateral sacral sensory loss and autonomic dysfunction. Numbness over dorsal medial foot and sole, weakness of ankle dorsiflexion and inversion. Impotence, bowel and bladder dysfunction possible. Patient may be unable to lie or sit down.
Leptomeningeal metastases (nerve root involvement) – Diffuse, multifocal involvement of subarachnoid, space by metastatic tumour. Non-Hodgkin's lymphoma and acute lymphocytic leukaemia most common. Breast and lung most common solid tumours. **Note:** CSF examination confirms diagnosis Gandolinium-enhanced CT/MRI for evaluation	Constant headache common, meningism may be present. Low back and buttock pain occur. Paroxysmal headache and other changes in mental/physical status may occur (lethargy, confusion, memory impairment). Nausea and vomiting may accompany pain. Multifocal neurological signs from all levels of neuraxis possible. Associated with very poor prognosis when untreated: often associated with other advanced disease.

Remember: An adequate trial of opioids should always be given first and the opioid continued with other techniques if the pain is partially opioid responsive.

INCIDENT PAIN

If there is no available cause-directed treatment (such as internal fixation) available, and if a trial of primary analgesics (NSAIDs and opioids) is ineffective, then intraspinal analgesia may be useful. Incident pain can be neuropathic, in full or in part, and the approach outlined above may help.

If neuropathic or incident pains do not respond to initial management early advice should be sought from a pain management clinic, so that a more specialized technique can be considered.

PRACTICAL GUIDE TO OPIOID THERAPY

When a powerful opioid needs to be prescribed, remember:

- to make time to explain to the patient and family why you are choosing a drug like morphine, and to answer their questions and fears about it
- to anticipate and explain possible adverse drug reactions and treat them prophylactically when appropriate. The patient must be **encouraged to report** them.
- to ensure that other staff do not have misconceptions about morphine and why it is being used.

COMMON FEARS ABOUT MORPHINE

- **Morphine is addictive**. Opioids are commonly drugs of abuse but this is outside the medical setting. There is no evidence to suggest that opioids given for medical reasons cause addiction. Physical, but not psychological, dependence can develop but does not cause problems if any necessary dose reductions are made gradually.
- **The dose needs to be constantly increased**. After titration the morphine dose is commonly stable until disease progression occurs, when the dose can be increased to useful effect. Morphine doses often go down as well as up, and some patients come off morphine altogether. True pharmacological tolerance to morphine's analgesic effects is rare, and is overcome by increasing the dose.

- **If morphine is used too early there will be nothing available when the pain gets really bad**. There is no upper limit to the dose of morphine that can be prescribed to improve pain relief, so long as the benefits outweigh the adverse effects.
- **Morphine is only used for dying patients**. Morphine can be used for patients with nociceptive pain of any origin: it is a very good analgesic and patients can remain on it for years and live a normal life.
- **The use of morphine will shorten a patient's life**. On the contrary, there is evidence to suggest that adequate pain relief will lengthen life. Any drug inappropriately prescribed can be hazardous, but morphine is a very safe drug when used properly. It is possible that the former practice of only prescribing morphine for the dying patient has led to its misplaced association with imminent death.
- **Parenteral morphine is more effective than oral morphine**. If the patient can take drugs by mouth then an oral preparation should be used. There is no evidence to demonstrate that parenteral morphine is more effective than oral morphine in comparable doses, although it is often tried if all other options have failed. Intraspinal morphine may sometimes give relief where oral morphine has failed.

STARTING DOSE OF ORAL MORPHINE

This will be dependent on:

- whether the patient has been taking an opioid, in which case a starting dose can be calculated if the patient is to be changed to morphine (see below and Table 14.8). A patient on a combination containing a weak opioid, e.g. co-proxamol, will generally need 10 mg 4-hourly as a starting dose (two tablets of co-proxamol is equivalent to 6 mg morphine in chronic use)
- the patient's age – reduce the dose with advancing age. A frail woman of 80 may only need 2.5 mg 4-hourly, with 'as required' doses available
- the patient's renal, hepatic and respiratory function – it is necessary to reduce both the dose and the frequency of medication initially when these are impaired. Such a patient may only require 2.5 mg every 8 hours initially, with 'as required' doses available
- the patient's general condition – reduce dose with increasing frailty.

A patient starting morphine therapy needs frequent review during the first 12–48 hours and whenever the dose is changed. The 'as required' dose should be the same as the regular 4-hourly dose.

In hospital it is often easiest to start the patient on regular 4-hourly morphine, with 'as required' doses for breakthrough pain, and convert him or her to twice or once-daily modified-release morphine when the pain is controlled. In the community the increased convenience of the modified-release preparations may outweigh the advantages of the increased dose flexibility of normal-release morphine, even when pain is not yet fully controlled. Ask the following questions when reviewing a patient on morphine therapy.

Is the patient still in pain?

If so, an increase in dose is generally required, particularly if pain relief is good until shortly before the next 4-hourly dose is due.

It takes five half-lives of a drug (about 20 hours for normal-release morphine) before plasma levels reach a steady state; 24 hours after starting morphine the pain should be significantly improved if the correct dose is being used. If there has been no improvement it may be that the pain is not, or is only poorly, opioid responsive. An adequate trial of opioid implies that the dose has been increased until the pain is controlled or adverse drug effects (e.g. sedation) have made further increases impossible. An alternative opioid of equivalent efficacy may then be tried. If the likely aetiology of the pain is neuropathic secondary analgesics or alternative techniques may be used earlier.

Every 24 hours:

- add up the total dose of morphine that has been given (regular and 'as required' doses) to calculate the daily dose
- if the pain is controlled on that total dose, divide by six to give the 4-hourly dose and the 'as required' dose
- if the pain is not controlled increase both the regular and 'as required' doses of morphine.

> **Most cancer patients have one morphine-responsive pain or one that is at least partially responsive. Remember that most cancer patients have more than one pain.**

Is the patient sleepy or being very sick in spite of appropriate treatment?

Most patients will be a little sleepy after starting morphine or following an increase in dose, but most become tolerant to this within days. One-third of patients suffer from nausea and/or vomiting when opioids are started, but again most become tolerant to this effect and do not require treatment after the first week of therapy. If these side-effects persist and there is no other explanation (they may be a result of the advancing disease, for example) ask:

- '**Has the pain improved at all**?' It may be only partially opioid responsive or non-responsive. Secondary analgesics may be needed as well as or even instead of morphine.
- If it has, '**Does this patient require an alternative strong opioid**?' Patients differ in how susceptible they are to the adverse effects of the different opioids, and may fare better on another drug of equivalent efficacy. Alternatively, an opioid-sparing drug or a special technique may be helpful.

ADVERSE EFFECTS FROM OPIOIDS

All opioids can cause adverse effects. Table 14.7 shows how these are treated. They should be both anticipated and actively managed. If the patient does not know what to expect and has no means of alleviating the unwanted drug effects, which are often temporary, he or she may lose confidence in opioids, refuse to take them, and a valuable tool in pain management will be lost. Some unwanted effects of opioids, such as myoclonic jerks or 'high-dose morphine pain,' may only be managed by changing to another opioid or by dose reduction. Intraspinal opioids can sometimes overcome intolerable adverse drug effects.

Important: When patients start morphine they should start a (softener + stimulant) laxative, e.g. codanthrusate: there is great interindividual variation in the dose needed to keep defecation comfortable. Patients with bowel obstruction can only have a faecal softener, e.g. docusate.

Since an individual's response to both the analgesic and adverse effects of different opioids is unpredictable, if one strong opioid is not tolerated or is ineffectual then another should be tried. In some units opioids are routinely 'rotated' in an effort to avoid these problems. In practice the great majority of patients needing powerful analgesia can be managed successfully on morphine.

If a patient has 'difficult pain' that is not responding to standard therapies, do not delay trying different opioids in turn or alternative drugs: seek advice from a clinician experienced in pain management.

TABLE 14.7 Management of the unwanted effects of morphine

Symptom	*Causes*	*Management*
Respiratory depression	Direct effect on μ receptors in the pons and medulla: rate, depth and rhythm of respiration altered leading to CO_2 retention	**Titrate dose against pain.** i.v./s.c. naloxone + artificial ventilation rarely necessary
Nausea and vomiting	Due to stimulation of chemoreceptor trigger zone (central effect) and gastric stasis (peripheral effect).	Antiemetics: haloperidol 1.5–3 mg b.d. p.o. (CTZ) or metoclopramide 10–20 mg t.d.s.
Constipation	Direct effect on smooth muscle of GI tract	Regular dose of stimulant + softening laxative. Great range in dose needed for control of constipation
Sedation	Central effect of morphine	Reduce dose of morphine if feasible, titrate dose against the pain, consider trial of psychostimulant (e.g. dexamphetamine or methylphenidate) if all else fails
Movement-related nausea and vomiting	Vestibular stimulation	Cyclizine 50–100 mg p.o./s.c.
Urinary retention	Increased smooth muscle tone in urinary tract	Catheterization may be necessary
Pruritus	Histamine release in the skin	Oral antihistamine
Bronchoconstriction	Histamine release in the bronchial tree	i.v./i.m. antihistamine with a bronchodilator CHANGE TO ANOTHER OPIOID IMMEDIATELY
Psychomimetic effects	Dysphoria, hallucinations and nightmares	Haloperidol 3–5 mg nocte
Morphine-induced pain: with *high-dose i.v. and i.t.* administration	Accumulation of M3G, which is an antagonist of the analgesic effects of morphine	May need to switch to alternative opioid, e.g. methadone, for severe pain

ALTERNATIVE POWERFUL OPIOIDS

Examples: fentanyl, hydromorphone, methadone.

Fentanyl

This may be given transdermally and is rarely used intravenously in cancer pain. Transdermal administration must only be used when opioid requirements are stable as plasma concentrations are slow to rise and fall. This has two disadvantages:

- If the painful stimulus recedes respiratory depression is a danger
- If the pain increases rescue analgesia will be required, and since oral fentanyl is not available another opioid will be needed, either by mouth or parenterally. This is usually morphine.

The exact indications for fentanyl in cancer pain are still being elucidated but it is certainly useful in some patients unable to take oral medication. It may be an alternative in patients who are susceptible to either the sedative or the constipating effects of morphine.

Methadone

Careful titration of methadone is essential for its safe and effective use. It cumulates in chronic dosing and its half-life is unpredictable (quoted figures are 8–80 hours), but the duration of its analgesia is only 4–8 hours. In the UK it is used as a second-line therapy. When converting a patient from methadone to morphine it is not helpful to calculate an equianalgesic dose (although this is often quoted as 1:1) as the requirement may be substantially lower. There are several suggested regimens for starting a patient on this drug – it is absolutely essential to keep the patient under close medical supervision, being vigilant for respiratory depression and sedation, until a stable, effective dose is reached.

Hydromorphone

This became available in the UK during 1997. It is reported to be an excellent analgesic with a short half-life and rapid onset of action. It may prove useful in patients unable to take morphine and in the frail elderly patient.

Changing opioid

When it is necessary to switch from one opioid to another, or from one route of administration to another, great care must be taken in calculating the required dose. Table 14.8 shows equianalgesic doses equivalent to 10 mg of morphine for some commonly used opioids.

TABLE 14.8 Equianalgesic doses of opioids with morphine

	Dose equianalgesic to morphine 10 mg i.m. (mg)		*Oral potency ratio*	
Drug	*i.m.*	*p.o.*	*Multiply oral dose of opioid by potency ratio to calculate oral equivalent dose of morphine sulphate*	*Duration of analgesia (h)*
Morphine-like agonists				
Morphine	10	30–60	1	3–6
Hydromorphone	1.5	7.5	8	3–5
Oxycodone		20–30	4/3	5–6
Pethidine	75	–	1/8	2–4
Diamorphine	3–5	–		4–5
Fentanyl (transdermal)	see drug data sheet	see drug data sheet	150	48–72
Codeine	130	200	1/10	3–5
Tramadol	100	–	1/4	5–6
Partial agonists				
Buprenorphine	0.3	0.8 (SL)	60	6–8

When converting from one opioid to another the dose of opioid in use can be multiplied by the quoted potency ratios to give a reasonable starting dose of oral morphine, but it should be remembered that:

- the dose of morphine may need to be higher or lower than the calculated one. Take into account the patient's renal function, age and frailty, and his or her reaction to the previous opioid
- in general the initial dose should be about 25% lower than the calculated one, because of incomplete cross-tolerance between opioid drugs
- if the patient was in pain on the previous opioid the dose of the new opioid should be higher than the calculated equianalgesic dose
- all conversions are approximate: start low and titrate up

Methadone is discussed in Chapter 3.

Converting to oral morphine from another opioid

Calculate the usual dose of opioid taken in a 24-hour period in milligrams – remember to include 'as required' doses.
Multiply this by the **relative potency** of the opioid in question (see Table 14.8). This will give the total daily dose of morphine that should give comparable relief.
If pain control has been unsatisfactory then the total daily dose of morphine should be increased by 30–50%.
If using normal-release morphine tablets or solution, divide the total by six to give the 4-hourly starting dose and 'as required' dose. This may need to be rounded up to the nearest 5 or 10 mg.
If using modified release morphine, divide by two and round up to the nearest convenient twice-daily dose. Divide the total by six to give the 'as required' dose.

BREAKTHROUGH PAIN

When a patient is started on regular morphine an 'as required' dose **equivalent to** the regular 4-hourly dose should be prescribed. Pain is the physiological antagonist of respiratory depression, and a patient in pain needs more analgesia. It is accepted practice to prescribe the 'as required' dose '1 hourly.'

If the patient is using modified-release morphine twice daily, add up the total daily dose and divide by six to give the 4-hourly equivalent dose and hence the 'as required' dose of morphine required.

Modified-release preparations are not suitable for use in breakthrough pain.

Increasing the dose

Dose adjustments should be large enough to make a difference within 24 hours. At lower doses the percentage increase will be higher.

A suggested regimen, in milligrams of morphine, is:

5→10→15→20→30→40→60→90/100→120/160→200/240→300/400 mg

ACUTE-ON-CHRONIC PAIN

Cancer patients on regular opioid therapy who have acute-on-chronic pain will need more than their equivalent daily opioid dose. Titrate the dose against the pain if such patients need surgery or a painful procedure.

TABLE 14.9 Calculating the dose of morphine and diamorphine required by different routes

Manoeuvre	*Necessary calculation*
Oral morphine to i.v. morphine	Divide by 3
Oral morphine to i.m./s.c. morphine	Divide by 2
Oral morphine to s.c. diamorphine	Divide by 3
Oral morphine to epidural morphine	Divide by 10
Oral morphine to intrathecal morphine	Divide by 100
Oral morphine to oral diamorphine	Nearly equivalent in chronic use

Whether converting between different opioid drugs or between different routes of administration, it is vital to keep the patient under review because of the known variability both in patients' rate of metabolism of these compounds and susceptibility to their analgesic and adverse effects. Calculated doses may have to be increased or decreased.

MONITORING PAIN

Pain measurement techniques have been discussed in Chapter 9. Many are too involved for routine clinical use, but when a large team is looking after a patient and the pain is changing it is helpful for the patient to keep a short, simple record of pain intensity to monitor the effectiveness of treatment. A brief pain diary, serial visual analogue scale (VAS) measurements or a simple verbal rating scale (pain mild, moderate or severe) can be used for these purposes. The record should be completed by the patient: pain ratings made by staff and relatives have been proved inaccurate.

USE OF A SYRINGE DRIVER

If the patient cannot take oral medication a continuous subcutaneous infusion of morphine, diamorphine or hydromorphone can be used so that 4-hourly injections are not required. In many instances other drugs will have to be used as well, and the greater solubility of diamorphine is useful here as the volume of injectate is reduced.

Drugs are continuously infused and are most often prescribed over a 24-hour period. There are many different models of syringe driver in use and when reviewing patients it is important to ensure that the prescribed dose is being accurately delivered.

A syringe driver is not a barrier to domiciliary care.

Enormous advances in cancer pain therapy have been achieved in the last 30 years. It is possible to give honest reassurance that most patients with cancer pain can be successfully managed on drugs alone.

Drugs should be given regularly, by mouth whenever possible, and using a methodical, systematic approach to the choice of agent or pain therapy technique. Regular pain therapy needs to be continued for as long as it is needed. Help is available whenever needed from palliative care specialists and pain clinic physicians – do not delay in seeking it.

CHAPTER 15

PAIN AND ADVANCED HIV DISEASE

INTRODUCTION

There has so far been little research completed on pain and HIV disease, but the available literature confirms that pain is both common and undertreated in patients with this condition. Quoted prevalence rates vary from 50 to 60% in hospice and hospital in-patients, to about 70% for patients at home. Pain becomes more common as death approaches. Patients with HIV disease are not commonly treated outside their specialist centres, because of both the complex nature of the drug regimens needed to manage the illness and the particular social problems associated with this diagnosis. Any new therapies should be instituted in consultation with the acute centre or hospice at which the patient is being primarily treated.

PATHOPHYSIOLOGY OF PAIN IN HIV DISEASE

The common pain syndromes involve:

- the gastrointestinal (GI) tract
- the central nervous system (CNS)
- the musculoskeletal system.

It is common for multiple pathological processes to cause pain in one patient.

The GI tract

The painful mouth and pharynx

Oral candidiasis. This occurs in up to 75% of HIV-positive people. The infection is not usually confined to the mouth and affects the pharynx and oesophagus as well. Although it may be asymptomatic candidiasis is also the commonest cause of pain in the mouth. The oesophagus may be affected when the mouth is not. It should be treated with systemic antifungal agents.

Mouth ulcers. There are several infectious agents that commonly cause mouth ulceration. These include herpes simplex virus, cytomegalovirus (CMV), Epstein–Barr virus, mycobacteria, cryptococcus and histoplasmosis. They may also infect the oesphagus as well. Idiopathic aphthous ulcers are also common in HIV disease.

Bacterial infections may also cause necrotizing gingivitis, and dental abscesses are also more common than in the general population.

Pain caused by infection should be treated symptomatically and with appropriate specific therapy.

Oesophagus. Pain and difficulty on swallowing is a problem for about one-third of patients with AIDS. The viral and bacterial infections which affect the mouth may be responsible (see above), and so is idiopathic ulceration.

Rare causes include neoplasia such as Kaposi's sarcoma and non-Hodgkin's lymphoma (NHL), but these are more likely to cause dysphagia alone.

The rest of the GI tract may be affected by infections and their complications (for example, intestinal perforation may occur secondary to CMV infection), Kaposi's sarcoma and NHL.

Pain associated with neurological disease

HIV is a neurotropic virus and affects both the peripheral and central nervous systems: one paper reported that 75% of patients with AIDS had neuropathological abnormalities at autopsy, 40% had significant neurological symptoms in life, and 10% had presented with neurological disease. Headache is very common in HIV disease. Make a careful diagnosis, and use any possible cause-directed treatment, as well as symptomatic relief.

Peripheral neuropathy

A symmetrical, mostly sensory, painful peripheral neuropathy is most commonly seen in patients with advanced HIV disease. Patients present with burning pain in the soles of their feet and paresthesiae which usually involve both the sole and the dorsum of the foot.

There may be a superimposed dull aching component to the pain. Mobility is often limited as the pain is exacerbated by weight-bearing. On examination patients will have decreased or absent ankle jerks and blunting of pain and vibration sense. The symptoms often remain confined to the glove and stocking distribution, although more formal testing will reveal that the signs have progressed beyond these limits.

Treatment

Peripheral neuropathy is often only partially opioid responsive and a tricyclic is often needed to achieve better control. TENS (see Chapter 8) was found helpful in one series.

Polyradiculopathies

Radicular pain is caused by CMV infection. The onset is slow but the syndrome is progressive: it typically begins with sacral and lumbar nerve root involvement, later affecting faecal and urinary continence.

Musculoskeletal pain

Arthritis, arthralgias and myopathies of various aetiologies are commonly associated with advanced HIV disease. Treatment is both symptomatic and specific.

Treatment strategies

The principles of treating pain associated with HIV disease are no different from those for treating cancer pain outlined in Chapter 14.

- Symptomatic treatment can begin before a diagnosis is made and specific therapy initiated.
- Assessment and treatment of the whole patient is vital for good pain management.
- For chronic pain pharmacological therapy needs to be given regularly, by mouth wherever possible.
- The WHO guidelines for cancer pain therapy provide a systematic approach to drug treatment for symptom control.
- Adjuvant drugs should be used where indicated (see below).
- Cause-directed treatment must be given as appropriate to the patient's general condition.
- Assessment by occupational and physotherapists and the provision of appropriate equipment (e.g. mattresses) and appliances is very important.
- Complementary therapies are often used for patients with HIV disease: evidence to define their indications and efficacy has not so far been collected.

Steroids should be used with great caution in these patients, who are already immunosuppressed. Specialist advice should be sought first.

A proportion of pain in HIV disease is associated with infection by other viruses and bacteria, and this requires specialist assessment and specific treatment. Symptomatic therapy can, however, begin immediately.

Undertreatment of pain

It has been amply demonstrated that pain in patients with advanced HIV disease is undertreated, the more severe the pain the greater the undertreatment. Many of the factors that contribute to the inadequate treatment of cancer pain seem to be responsible (see Chapter 14), but there are some studies which have identified factors particular to HIV disease.

Clinicians' unfamiliarity with opioids

HIV disease is treated by specialists who may have received little training in pain therapy. This may contribute to their reluctance to prescribe strong opioids, which have been found to be both effective and well tolerated in these patients.

Intravenous drug users

Intravenous drug abuse is associated with HIV disease, and most surveys have found that this subgroup of patients receives particularly poor pain control. It has been suggested that patients taking oral methadone as part of their treatment strategy for drug abuse are reluctant to use it at increased doses for pain relief. Drug abuse is associated with poverty, and this is another identified risk factor for receiving inadequate analgesia.

Dementia

A large proportion of patients with advanced HIV disease suffer from dementia. This may make pain assessment and control more difficult.

Poverty

It has been shown that those patients who are poor (particularly if they have a low IQ) are more likely to receive inadequate pain therapy.

SECTION 4

CHRONIC PAIN SYNDROMES

CHAPTER 16

BACK AND NECK PAIN

BACK PAIN

INTRODUCTION

The management of low back pain, with or without lower limb symptoms, forms the bulk of practice in most pain clinics (80% in the author's clinic). The spectrum of presentation is wide. The pain clinician may be the first specialist that the patient sees, and therefore diagnosis and appropriate investigation must be organized. Alternatively, patients may have had multiple imaging investigations and operations and management of their pain presents a different challenge.

Low back pain is very common: up to 80% of adults will experience back pain at some time. Around 80% of episodes are self-limiting within 2 weeks. Of those seeking medical attention the majority will not receive a definitive diagnosis. Recent figures suggest a total working incapacity of 150 million days per year attributable to back pain, with a total cost to the NHS of around £480 million. These figures are increasing yearly. It is important to emphasise that it is low back disability which is increasing so rapidly, and not necessarily an increase in the incidence of low back pain. In countries without sophisticated healthcare provision the incidence of back-related disability is much lower.

AETIOLOGY

There is little correlation between pathological processes, symptoms, signs and imaging investigations. It is as important to address the impact of the pain on the patient's life as to attend to the anatomical source of the problem (which may be impossible to define). Many structures have been described as giving rise to low back pain, but in practice the aim is to exclude a number of specific conditions (which make up a small proportion of the back pain population):

- Underlying systemic disease
- Infection
- Malignancy
- Unrecognized trauma
- Neurological compromise, nerve root damage, spinal stenosis, cauda equina syndrome.

Most patients presenting to the pain clinic will fall into one of three categories:

- Non-specific 'mechanical' low back pain
- Nerve root compromise
- Postsurgical back pain.

MECHANICAL BACK PAIN

This is a non-specific diagnosis and usually implies pain arising from posterior elements in the spine. Pain may be confined to the lumbar spine but may be referred to the groin or lower limbs. It is **uncommon** for pain to radiate below the knee (see below). Signs of root dysfunction cannot be demonstrated. Many structures may give rise to mechanical back pain, but the facet joints and muscles are the most common therapeutic targets.

Facet joints

The facet joints are synovial joints (Figure 16.1) with a joint space, hyaline cartilage surfaces, synovial membrane and a fibrous capsule. They can undergo the inflammatory and degenerative changes of rheumatoid or osteoarthritis and the ligamentous and capsular pathologies similar to peripheral joints. The joints carry loads via lumbar extension, and this is increased in the presence of degenerative disc disease or following disc surgery. The facet joint capsule is richly innervated and hence capsular deformation is potentially painful. Pain is typically felt in the back, radiating into the posterior thigh. (**NB.** as the joints are supplied by the posterior primary rami of the spinal nerves, the pain may be referred by the anterior primary rami of the same nerves and be experienced in the leg.) There is often a history of morning stiffness. On examination, pressure over the facet joints is painful. Straight leg raising (see below) is normal and neurological examination is often unremarkable.

Degenerative facet joint disease is a frequent finding in all types of imaging of the lumbar spine, our treatments directed at the facet joints or their nerve supply often have disappointing results.

Muscles of the back

The significance of muscle as a source of low back pain is unclear. Muscles contain a large population of Aδ and C fibres, a proportion of which serve a nociceptive function. Examination of patients with back pain often reveals muscle spasm or tender trigger points, nodules and bands. Attention to these trigger areas can occasionally produce dramatic relief of back pain symptoms.

SPINAL INSTABILITY

The definition of spinal instability is controversial. Instability is generally described as the inability of supporting structures of the spine to resist physiologic loads, thereby permitting abnormal spinal movement sufficient to cause pain. Symptoms usually include pain radiating to the buttocks and upper thighs or inguinal and abductor regions (rarely radiating below the knees). Bilateral symptoms are common. Pain is exacerbated by movement and may be associated with a 'catching sensation'. Coughing and straining do

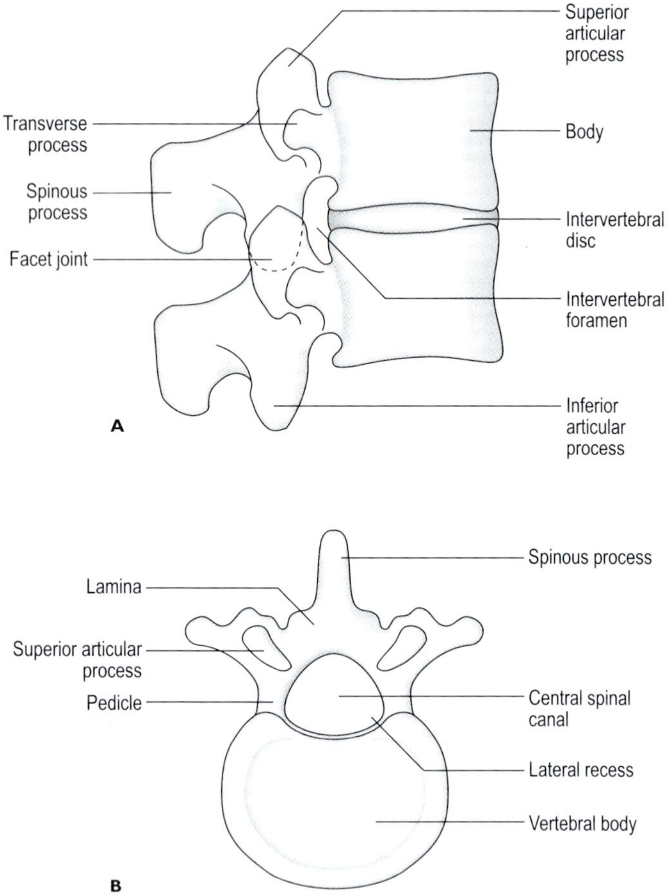

Fig. 16.1 (**a**) Lateral and (**b**) transverse views of lumbar vertebrae.

not exacerbate symptoms. Clinical signs vary. There may be an exaggerated lumbar lordosis and there is often diffuse tenderness over the involved segments. The range of spinal motion may be full. Signs of root tension are usually absent. Surgical management of spinal instability is considered below.

NERVE ROOT COMPROMISE

Nerve root compromise may result from a prolapsed intervertebral disc or degenerative bony and ligamentous overgrowth. Individual nerve roots may be affected or the cauda equina may become compressed.

The lumbar nerve roots leave the vertebral canal via the intervertebral foramen (IVF) (see Figure 16.1). The anterior boundaries of the IVF comprise the vertebral bodies and end plates, the intervertebral disc and the posterior longitudinal ligament. The foramen is bordered posteriorly by the facet joints, pars interarticularis, pedicles and ligamentum flavum. The upper lumbar nerve roots pass out almost at a right-angle from the dural sac, whereas the lower roots have a longer intraspinal course before passing through the IVF. The lumbar nerve roots may be compressed *anteriorly* by disc protrusion/herniation and accompanying osteophyte formation, and *posteriorly* by degenerate hypertrophied facet joints and ligamentum flavum.

Compression of normal nerve roots does not cause pain, but if the nerve root is inflamed and irritated (as occurs with chronic compression) then pain will occur. A herniated disc can also impinge on the dorsal root ganglion, which is exquisitely sensitive to mechanical pressure. In addition, some pain may be referred from distortion of neighbouring muscle insertions, joint capsules and ligaments.

Disc lesions

The intervertebral disc is attached to the vertebral end plates superiorly and inferiorly and to the anterior and posterior longitudinal ligaments. It comprises a central ovoid mass of gelatinous material under pressure – the nucleus pulposus. With advancing age the water content of the nucleus pulposus decreases and is replaced by fibrocartilage. The nucleus pulposus is surrounded by the fibrocartilaginous annulus fibrosus. This is made up of concentric layers of collagen fibres which pass obliquely between adjacent vertebral bodies, and is strongly attached to the anterior and posterior longitudinal ligaments. Degenerative disease predisposes to disc prolapse (peak incidence between 30 and 55 years). A tear develops in the annulus fibrosus and a fragment of the nucleus herniates posteriorly into the defect, causing root compromise in the spinal canal or IVF.

Spinal stenosis (bony entrapment)

Degenerative overgrowth of the vertebral bodies, facet joints and ligamentum flavum can cause nerve root entrapment, either alone or in addition to disc herniation. Stenosis may be in the central canal, the lateral recess or the root canal. Combinations of the above may exist.

Central stenosis

Pain may be felt in the low back, buttocks and legs. It is diffuse and aching in nature and the lower limbs may feel heavy. Extension of the spine exacerbates the pain and flexion eases it (walking uphill is easier than on the flat). It is important to differentiate this condition from vascular claudication.

Lateral recess stenosis

The pain tends to occur in a radicular distribution. Sensory symptoms and examination findings may be confusing. The condition may be self-limiting but around 10% of patients may require surgery.

Cauda equina syndrome

Acute compression of the cauda equina is rare. It is caused by a large disc herniation, usually in the midline, impinging on the S2 and lower nerve roots. It is characterized by loss of bladder and bowel sphincter control and saddle-shaped loss of sensation in sacral dermatomes. Unilateral or bilateral sciatica with impaired straight leg raising may be noted. The condition constitutes a surgical emergency.

POSTSURGICAL BACK PAIN

It is difficult to quantify success rates for spinal surgery, which depend critically on the indications for surgery. It is probably safe to say that primary surgery for lumbar disc herniation in well selected patients who have good concordance between history, examination findings and the results of imaging tests performs better than in other patients who have surgery for non-specific pain conditions. However, a significant proportion of back pain patients presenting to the pain clinic have persisting pain following surgery. Increasingly strict operative criteria and improved imaging of the lumbar spine should help reduce the problem.

There may be an obvious cause for persisting symptoms:

- Wrong operation (wrong diagnosis/wrong level)
- Infection
- Technical complication (CSF fistula etc.)
- Recurrent disc herniation
- Presence of coincidental pathology.

In general decompressive operations to relieve leg pain do not alleviate back pain, and may exacerbate it.

Disc surgery results in increasing stress on the neighbouring facet joints, enhancing degenerative disease and giving rise to the typical symptoms of posterior compartment pain. Repeated surgery is likely to result in epidural fibrosis and root scarring. A proportion of patients will develop adhesive arachnoiditis, in which damage to the pia mater of the cauda equina results in constricting fibrous bands around nerve tissue. Treatment is notoriously difficult and psychological sequelae from the unrelenting pain are common.

Many patients who have been appropriately selected and who have technically successful operations without complications still have persistent pain. Certainly if there has been prolonged nerve damage prior to surgery it is likely that permanent peripheral and central changes have taken place in the nervous system which prolong and enhance the pain experience.

ASSESSMENT OF THE PATIENT WITH BACK PAIN

HISTORY

At the initial consultation the pain should be characterized in the way described in Chapter 9. When assessing lumbar spine problems it is important to ascertain whether symptoms are predominantly in the back, the leg(s) or both. Pain from discs, facet joints and ligaments is felt in the lower back, often radiating to the SI joints, buttocks, groin, hip and thigh. It is unusual for such back pain to radiate below the knee. The history must be sufficient to exclude serious spinal pathology or underlying systemic disease (although this will usually have been detected before referral to the pain clinic).

NB: Back pain may be caused by visceral disease, e.g. of pelvic organs, kidneys, GI tract and aorta.

Features in the history which suggest serious spinal pathology are summarized in Table 16.1.

The history will also aid diagnosis of neurological compromise (Table 16.2).

EXAMINATION

The behaviour of the patient can be observed as he or she walks to the consulting room. The presence and appropriateness of aids (sticks, crutches etc.) should be noted. Patients may have difficulty in sitting throughout the consultation, and should be invited to stand or move around. Formal examination should include inspection of the back, noting abnormal posture and, in particular, kyphosis, scoliosis or loss of lumbar lordosis. Palpation may reveal spinal or paraspinal tenderness or muscle spasm with trigger points.

TABLE 16.1 Features in history suggesting serious spinal pathology

Pathology	*Features in history*
Malignancy (accounts for less than 1% episodes of back pain)	Age – over 50 in 80% cases Previous history of malignancy Unexplained weight loss Progressive symptoms unresponsive to simple treatments Failure of bed rest to relieve symptoms
Infection	Obvious source, e.g. indwelling urinary catheter, skin infections, history of i.v. drug abuse, HIV, TB Systemically unwell
Fracture	History of trauma Long-term steroid therapy (osteoporosis – commonest in age >70)
Ankylosing spondylitis and other inflammatory arthritides	High sensitivity and specificity if four positive answers out of: (1) morning stiffness? (2) Improvement with excercise? (3) Onset <40(4) Slow onset? (5) Pain persisting >3 months? Family history Widespread persisting limitation of spinal movement Peripheral joint involvement Associated phenomena (iritis, rashes, colitis, urethritis)

TABLE 16.2 Symptoms of neurological compromise

Type of neurological involvement	*Symptoms*
Nerve root pain (most commonly lumbar disc herniation – commonly ages 30–55 – but also entrapment by bony/ligamentous hypertrophy)	Unilateral leg pain > back pain (usually radiates to foot, exacerbated by sneezing/coughing/Valsalva Numbness and paraesthesia (same distribution) Weakness
Spinal stenosis	Usually age >55 Long history Neurogenic claudication (pain in legs on walking) Better on flexion – patient can often cycle Exacerbated by sneezing/coughing
Cauda equina syndrome	Urinary retention Faecal incontinence Anaesthesia around perineum/genitals Weakness of legs/alteration in gait

Mobility of the lumbar spine may be assessed by asking the patient to bend forward. Pain on extension should be noted. Formally assess lateral flexion and rotation. With the patient standing it is useful to ask him to stand on his heels (L5 function) and toes (S1 function).

With the patient supine on the couch straight leg raising (SLR) should be measured. This assesses tension in the lower lumbar nerve roots. The heel is cupped in the examiner's hand and the patient's leg raised from the couch with the knee extended. If buttock or leg (not back) pain is elicited when the leg is raised (particularly if this is exacerbated on dorsiflexion of the foot), this suggests nerve root tension. A more specific test is crossed SLR, which elicits pain in the affected leg on raising the contralateral limb. Tension on the L3 and L4 roots can be assessed by the femoral stretch test. The patient lies prone and the affected leg is flexed at the knee. Pain in the anterior thigh suggests root tension.

The results of formal sensory testing should be documented, and although it is useful to remember the appropriate dermatomes in the lower limb it is important to remember that they are not constant from individual to individual, and that dermatomal charts differ. Nerve root compromise usually presents with sensory loss in a dermatomal pattern. Muscle power and deep tendon reflexes must also be assessed (Table 16.3).

TABLE 16.3 Root values of tendon reflexes and muscle groups in the lower limb

Neurological sign	*Corresponding root*
Power	
Quadriceps	L4
Extensor hallucic longus	L5
Plantar flexors	S1
Reflexes	
Knee jerk	L4
Ankle jerk	S1

The importance of documenting neurological signs cannot be overemphasized. A change in neurological findings may represent disease progression.

IMAGING OF THE LUMBAR SPINE

Plain X-rays

These are not necessary for every patient with low back pain. Radiography of the lumbar spine involves relatively high radiation doses and there is a low yield of useful findings and a wide variation in interpretation between clinicians, even in the same specialty. Pain correlates poorly with changes found on X-ray.

Patients with a first episode of low back pain of less than 7 weeks' duration who are untreated or improving with treatment do not need X-rays of the lumbar spine. Exceptions are:

- Age under 20 or over 55
- Presence of neurological deficit (including urinary tract dysfunction)
- Evidence of infection (fever etc.)
- Suspicion of malignancy (history of cancer, weight loss)
- Systemic steroids
- Drug abuse
- Obvious structural deformity
- History of trauma
- Progressive pain unresponsive to treatment.

AP and lateral X-rays will usually be sufficient.

X-rays may be normal in the presence of serious spinal pathology, e.g. early infection/tumour.

Computed tomography (CT)

Although it gives more detail than plain radiographs and defines bony anatomy well, CT is unreliable in the diagnosis of disc lesions. CT myelography is a useful alternative in patients who are unable to tolerate MRI scanning or are excluded from it by the presence of spinal instrumentation.

Magnetic resonance imaging (MRI)

This is currently the gold standard in the investigation of spinal disorders. Results should be interpreted with the knowledge that single or multilevel degeneration or disc bulge is visible in between 28 and 85% of the adult population (both sexes) who do not have activity-limiting low back pain (i.e. it has low specificity). The prevalence of abnormal findings rises with age. MRI is, however, highly sensitive. **Findings on MRI must not be considered**

to be causally related to the patient's symptoms without confirmation from physical signs on examination. MRI with gadolinium enhancement is particularly useful in patients following surgery, as it helps distinguish fibrosis from persisting disc fragments.

MANAGEMENT OF BACK PAIN

ACUTE BACK PAIN

Over 80% of episodes of low back pain will settle within 2 weeks. The early management is important in encouraging recovery and preventing chronicity. The aim of management is to control symptoms while spontaneous recovery occurs. The pain can usually be managed by the patient with advice from his general practitioner. The cornerstones of management are simple oral analgesics and encouragement to mobilize.

Medication

In the first few days of the back pain episode it may be helpful to take medication on a regular timed basis, rather than PRN. First-line drugs include paracetamol and NSAIDs, e.g. ibuprofen, both of which are available without prescription. Topical NSAIDs may also provide good symptomatic relief. It may be necessary to provide compound minor opioid preparations for a few days.

Exercise

Bed rest is no longer considered appropriate in the management of simple acute back pain as it encourages immobility and leads to stiffness and symptoms of muscle disuse. In general, patients should be advised to keep as mobile as possible. Active exercise such as walking, cycling and swimming should be encouraged, with activity being increased in a graded manner. Patients with simple back pain must understand that they will not harm themselves by being active. Simple manipulation may be beneficial at this early stage.

If after 6 weeks, these simple measures fail diagnosis should be reviewed and psychological and social factors which may be perpetuating the pain should be explored.

CHRONIC BACK PAIN

Because the causes of back pain are multifactorial it is unsurprising that there is no universally successful treatment. In reality, most patients presenting to the pain clinic will receive most types of treatment, with the order in which they are delivered being dictated by the presenting symptoms. Treatments may be categorized as follows:

- Medication
- Stimulation techniques
- Injections
- Physical therapy
- Psychological treatment
- Surgery.

Medication therapy is summarized in Table 16.4.

TABLE 16.4 Medication in the management of low back pain

Medication	*Comments*
Simple oral analgesics	
Compound minor opioids	Patients will usually have tried maximum doses of these drugs to no good effect, but they are reluctant to stop them. If the drugs are genuinely not helping they should be discontinued. The maximum dose is limited by the paracetamol content of the tablets. Occasionally worth changing to regular rather than PRN dosing
NSAIDs	Useful drugs, especially for morning stiffness. Most patients will have tried them. It is important to take a full drug history to ascertain whether the patient has taken an appropriate dose for long enough to assess effect. Reasons for discontinuation of the drug must be noted: if because of gastric side-effects it may be worth trying NSAID/misoprostol combination or selective COX2 inhibitor. Worth trying a number of different preparations e.g. diclofenac SR 75 mg once/twice daily, or indomethacin SR 75 mg once/twice daily
Tricyclic antidepressants	Logical drugs if suspect nerve damage component of pain. Sedative side-effects useful in patients who sleep poorly because of pain
Anticonvulsants	Use in neuralgic pain well defined. May be helpful in cases of nerve root dysfunction with typical neuropathic features (e.g. in presence of root scarring)

Stimulation techniques

TENS

This is widely used in the treatment of back pain. Most patients will try this safe therapy as it allows them to control their own treatment. It may be particularly useful if the patient has a significant myofascial component.

Acupuncture

This may be a useful therapy, especially in the presence of muscle spasm.

Dorsal column stimulation

The literature on the efficacy of dorsal column stimulation is anecdotal. The commonest diagnostic group, which has been repeatedly described, are patients with continuing back pain following surgery, particularly those with nerve root scarring, epidural fibrosis and adhesive arachnoiditis. Published series in these patients suggest improved activities of daily living, reduction in medication and satisfaction with treatment. Properly controlled trials are needed.

Injection therapy

Epidural

The value of injecting local anaesthetic and steroid into the epidural space remains controversial, but the technique is widely used. Disc injury is associated with propagation of an inflammatory cascade via arachidonic acid liberation. Similar inflammatory processes have been described in the presence of nerve root compression. Steroids have a number of anti-inflammatory properties, hence the rationale for their use. In addition they have inhibitory effects on C-fibre conduction, which may account for part of their action. Injection of these drugs into the epidural space allows a higher local concentration than systemic administration, which would depend on epidural blood flow to reach its target site (this may be reduced in the presence of root compression).

Most clinicians co-administer local anaesthetic with the steroid, because it makes the injection more comfortable and it may interrupt the sustained abnormal neural activity that perpetuates the pain.

There is little agreement about:

- the dose or type of steroid to be used
- the dose or type of local anaesthetic
- the need for combined local anaesthetic and steroid
- the route of epidural injection (caudal, lumbar translaminal, transforaminal)
- the volume of injectate
- the frequency of injections.

Recent controversy has arisen over the use of Depo-Medrone (methylprednisolone). Reports of its intrathecal use in Australia suggested that the polyethylene glycol used as a dispersant may have contributed to the development of arachnoiditis. No such complications have been reported in large series of epidural Depo-Medrone. Many clinicians now prefer to use triamcinolone, which does not contain polyethylene glycol. **As with the use of any non-licensed drug it is advisable to explain to the patient, when**

asking them to sign the consent form that steroids are not licensed for epidural use.

The complications of epidural injection are usually transient and include headache, backache and leg pain. Inadvertent dural puncture occurs in 0.5–2.5% of patients. Although the caudal route minimizes this complication, the incidence of misplacement of the injection (i.e. outside the epidural space) rises.

Data regarding efficacy are conflicting. Many of the existing randomized trials of epidural injection are methodologically flawed. Most studies suggest that patients with compressive lumbar radiculopathy do better than those with lumbosacral pain alone. Further rigorously controlled trials are necessary to determine the benefits of this frequently used treatment.

Facet joint procedures

The lumbar facet joints may be a source of low back pain. Injection of local anaesthetic and/or steroid into the joint or its nerve supply may provide pain relief, and the anatomical accessibility of the facet joints has led this to become a popular technique.

Injections. Injection of the joints should be conducted with X-ray screening. The volume of the joint is small and less than 2 ml is the recommended volume of injectate. A good response to sequential local anaesthetic blocks may confirm the facet joint as a source of pain. More usually the joint is injected with a combination of local anaesthetic and steroid (the latter for its anti-inflammatory effect). Usually the L3/4, L4/5 and L5/S1 joints are injected bilaterally.

Denervation. Pain relief may be achieved by the injection of local anaesthetic and/or steroid in the region of the posterior primary ramus which supplies the joint. They are injected at the junction of the transverse process and the pedicle of the appropriate lumbar vertebra. Effective but transient relief from facet joint injection or pharmacological denervation may suggest that long-term analgesia can be achieved by radiofrequency or cryotherapeutic destruction of the posterior primary ramus, but this is not always the case. The innervation of the facet joint is complex, and therefore it is unsurprising that destruction of the posterior primary ramus does not always result in pain relief.

The efficacy of facet joint injections is debated in the literature. Studies show no consistent difference between any of the following: intra-articular and periarticular injection; posterior primuary ramus blocks or denervations; use of local anaesthetic, local anaesthetic and steroid or injection of saline. Similarly, there are no conclusive studies suggesting good predictors of outcome for such procedures. Empirical observation suggests that some patients improve following facet joint procedures, but further research is needed to evaluate outcomes from different techniques and to optimize patient selection.

Physical therapy

Physical exercise, and more particularly the avoidance of immobility, should underpin other treatments for back pain. In a simple acute back pain exercise may be all that is required, but in more chronic cases it may be a useful adjunct to other therapies. It is common for patients to experience an initial increase in pain with exercise but they must be reassured that this is not harmful. There is evidence that exercise may improve disc nutrition and reduce the risk of recurrent back pain. Most chronic back pain patients have poor spinal musculature as a result of disuse (exacerbated by the use of corsets and lumbar spinal supports), and muscle strengthening excercises are likely to improve symptoms.

Psychological management

It is important to re-emphasize that many back pain patients have lived with their pain for years, and the impact of the pain on their lives is as important as the source of the pain (if known). The extent to which a patient is disabled by back pain depends on his or her beliefs about and attitudes to the pain. The pain clinic psychologist has much to offer these patients, particularly in the context of a multidisciplinary pain management programme (see Chapter 22).

Surgical management

There are few instances when surgery is indicated for back pain alone. The presence of neurologic compromise (diagnosed from history, physical signs and the results of imaging investigations) may be an indication for surgery. Even so, one retrospective study comparing conservative management of sciatica with surgical treatment showed no difference at 6-month follow-up. A large prospective study of patients with prolapsed intervertebral disc showed that 90% were symptomatically improved at 31 months without treatment. Back surgery rates vary between countries and are closely related to the per capita supply of neurosurgeons and orthopaedic surgeons.

Decisions regarding which type of surgery is appropriate for patients with low back pain (with or without lower limb symptoms) rest with specialist orthopaedic and neurosurgeons. The role of the non-surgical clinician is to select those patients who may need specialist referral and assessment. In order to do this it is useful to know what type of surgical techniques are available for managing these patients. Although improvements in imaging techniques have enhanced the ability to detect surgically remediable lesions in the lumbar spine, decisions on surgery should depend upon clinical symptoms and neurological signs, in addition to radiologic information. Procedures may be divided into three categories, summarized in Table 16.5.

TABLE 16.5 Surgical management of back pain

Procedure	*Comments*
Disc surgery	
Laminectomy	Formerly standard approach to prolapsed disc. Controversial procedure now abandoned in some spinal practice, except for large central discs with cauda equina syndrome. Being replaced by less invasive procedures
Microdiscectomy	Removes prolapsed free fragment only. Remaining disc is conserved, with minimal disruption of lumbar spinal architecture but higher risk of reprolapse. Removal of more disc minimizes reprolapse rate but distorts anatomy, with end plate collapse and increased strain on facet joints, often increasing postoperative back pain
Procedures for bony entrapment	
Intersegmental decompression	Involves removal of inferior and superior laminae, medial facetectomy and foraminotomy. Achieves the necessary decompression of spinal stenosis without marked disruption of spinal motion, as often occurs with laminectomy. Helps to diminish risks of instability. Used in cases of spinal stenosis with or without disc prolapse
Foraminotomy	Indicated when stenosis is in root canal, usually due to degenerative disease with osteophyte formation
Fusion procedures for spinal instability	Since definition and diagnosis not agreed the surgical method of fusion (bone grafting, instrumentation etc.) or the approach (posterior or anterior) probably less important than patient selection when determining outcome. Poor association between fusion solidity and pain relief

CONCLUSION

Many conditions presenting to the pain clinic have well worked out aetiologies, which allows a rational approach to diagnosis and management. Most pain-clinicians see far more patients who have back pain than any other chronically painful condition. Despite this, we still do not know why patients get back pain, and no hypothesis explains the huge range of symptoms that present. Pointers in the history may suggest a contributory anatomical source for pain, but all too frequently, therapy directed at the offending structure fails to provide relief. Patients are subjected to a range of procedures which do not have proven outcomes, and for many no improvement of symptoms is achieved. The most useful approach to management is multidisciplinary, as might be expected from the complexity of the condition. The therapy of back pain is an area where urgent research is needed so that appropriate therapy can be directed towards correctly selected patients who are likely to benefit from our efforts.

NECK PAIN

INTRODUCTION

Neck pain is common, affecting over one in ten of the adult population. There are many structures in the neck which may give rise to pain, including muscles, ligaments, facet joints, discs and non-spinal structures. It is important in the assessment of the patient with neck pain to exclude underlying systemic disease in the same way as described for those presenting with pain in the lumbar spine. In addition, it should be noted that meningeal irritation by infection or blood may present as neck pain (almost always acutely).

IMAGING OF THE CERVICAL SPINE

Plain X-rays of the cervical spine, including lateral films in flexion and extension, may give useful information about bony structures, including canal and foraminal narrowing. The atlantoaxial joint may be seen on an open-mouth view. Cervical spondylosis is an almost universal X-ray finding in the elderly population and is common in younger patients. The degree of spondylosis correlates poorly with pain symptoms. Myelography with CT scanning provides much more information about the nature of bony disease and demonstrates discs and neural structures well, but is being increasingly superseded by MRI. Again, MRI abnormalities, particularly osteophyte formation and disc protrusion, are common findings in neurologically asymptomatic individuals, particularly the elderly. All treatment decisions must be based on the triad of history, clinical examination findings and the results of imaging investigations.

CERVICAL SPONDYLOSIS

Degenerative disease of the cervical spine is very common. It is an almost universal radiological finding in those over the age of 50, but the majority of people are asymptomatic. As with the lumbar spine there is no correlation between X-ray findings and severity of symptoms. The C5/6 and C6/7 levels are the most commonly affected. Symptomatic individuals usually present with stiffness and decreased range of movement of the cervical spine. Neck pain is thought to arise from the facet joints. Treatment (in the absence of radiculopathy or myelopathy) is with simple oral analgesics (e.g. NSAIDs) in the first instance. Muscular trigger points can often be elicited and symptoms may improve with trigger point injections. Because of the suggested role of the facet joints in the genesis of the pain, cervical facet joint injections/denervations are considered useful. The role of cervical epidural injection in the absence of radiculopathy is controversial. TENS or acupuncture may be beneficial.

CERVICAL RADICULOPATHY

Cervical nerve roots may be compressed as a result of degenerative bony overgrowth or protrusion of disc material. Symptoms in the arm are similar to those in the lower limb following lumbar disc herniation, and include neck and arm pain (usually unilateral), sensory changes including paraesthesia, and weakness of the affected limb with hyporeflexia. The commonest levels for cervical disc prolapse are C5/6 and C6/7. Acute onset of symptoms suggests disc prolapse, whereas symptoms of slower onset are likely to be due to osteophyte formation. Spontaneous resolution of symptoms may occur. Non-operative treatments include cervical traction, physiotherapy and TENS. Helpful medications include NSAIDs, other simple oral analgesics, and tricyclic antidepressants and anticonvulsants if the pain is of neuropathic character. Decompressive surgery is indicated for recurrent motor and sensory symptoms, or failure of conservative measures to manage pain.

CERVICAL MYELOPATHY

Again, this condition may be caused by degenerative bony overgrowth or disc herniation. The symptoms may appear insidiously. The features are of upper motor neurone symptoms in the lower limbs, particularly gait disturbance and weakness and occasionally bladder dysfunction. Symptoms in the arms include tingling, weakness and clumsiness. Spasticity in all four limbs may be noted on examination. Myelopathy tends to be progressive, with little spontaneous improvement. Early decompressive surgery may resolve symptoms.

OCCIPITAL NEURALGIA

This term describes recurring pain in the upper neck and occipital region in the distribution of the greater occipital nerve, which is mostly a direct continuation of the posterior C2 root. It is most commonly seen in the presence of C1/2 spondylytic disease. The pain is usually described as prolonged (rather than paroxysmal), felt unilaterally mostly in the occiput, and radiating to the vertex or temporal region. The pain often has stabbing exacerbations, particularly on movement of the neck. On examination the nerve is often tender at the occiput and percussion may elicit paraesthesia in its distribution. Abnormal sensory phenomena may be noted. The condition usually responds to repeated occipital nerve block with local anaesthetic and depot steroid. Cryotherapy to the nerve produces longer-lasting analgesia. Pharmacological management includes the use of NSAIDs and antineuralgic drugs.

WHIPLASH INJURY

Considerable diagnostic confusion surrounds this term, but it most commonly describes the injury sustained in a motor vehicle accident where the head is subject to acceleration forces, usually following rear-end impact. The structures of the neck are subject to forced hyperextension followed by forward flexion. Unless the head is in the anatomical position and the force transmitted along the long axis of the vehicle, there will also be lateral flexion and rotation injury. This may result in damage to muscles, ligaments, facet joints and discs. The condition is common, probably occuring in around one-fifth of patients involved in a rear-end collision. It occurs most commonly in the third to fifth decades. Prevalence studies suggest no gender difference, but females are overrepresented in this condition compared to other motor vehicle injuries. Early symptoms include neck, shoulder and occipital pain, and less commonly headaches, visual disturbance, tinnitus and cognitive impairment. Physical signs include tenderness and reduced range of movement of the cervical spine. Neurological signs are found rarely and may suggest more severe damage. Imaging investigations are often unhelpful.

Most patients recover from whiplash injury. It is difficult to determine what proportion develop persistent symptoms (whiplash syndrome), but it is probably of the order of 10%. Persistent symptoms most commonly include neck pain, stiffness and headache. Sufferers exhibit abnormal psychological distress, but it is not known whether this is a consequence of the continuing pain.

Treatment of early whiplash has traditionally included simple oral analgesia, including NSAIDs, a cervical collar, physiotherapy, trigger point injections and TENS. It is not known to what extent these treatments alter the natural history of the condition. Treatments for chronic whiplash syndrome are not supported by good randomized controlled trials. Epidural steroid injections and cervical facet joint injections are frequently performed, but without rational basis. Similarly, the use of TENS and pharmacotherapy, including tricyclic antidepressants and anticonvulsants, has anecdotal support. Behavioural therapy in the context of a multidisciplinary pain management programme may help the patient cope more adequately with symptoms and improve function.

CHAPTER 17

MUSCULAR PAIN

INTRODUCTION

There are a number of chronic pain syndromes thought to arise from muscle. The most important of these are fibromyalgia syndrome (FMS) and myofascial pain syndrome (MPS). There are a number of common features between the two conditions.

FIBROMYALGIA SYNDROME

Fibromyalgia is a chronic pain disorder which is characterized by generalized muscular pain, the presence of tender points, stiffness and non-restorative sleep patterns. It occurs much more commonly in females than males (10:1) and usually between the ages of 30 and 50. Sensitive and specific criteria for the diagnosis of fibromyalgia have considerably enhanced identification of this condition (Table 17.1)

CLINICAL FEATURES

In addition to the diagnostic criteria a number of other features are common in FMS sufferers, notably fatigue, stiffness and non-restorative sleep pattern. Features of FMS may also develop in patients with autoimmune disease, e.g. rheumatoid arthritis, systemic lupus erythematosis, Raynaud's disease and hypothyroidism.

PAIN

Pain is generalized and usually described as a muscular ache. It tends to be persistent and pain sites remain unchanged. Pain and stiffness are more proximal than distal. The low back, neck, shoulders and hips are commonly reported sites for pain.

TENDER POINTS

Tender points are characteristic of fibromyalgia and are distinct from trigger points (see below). Palpation of tender points causes local pain, often described as severe. They are not associated with palpable nodules or bands in the muscle.

TABLE 17.1 The American College of Rheumatology 1990 criteria for the classification of fibromyalgia

1. History of widespread pain	Definition: pain is considered widespread when all of the following are present: pain in the left side of the body, pain in the right side of the body, pain above the waist, pain below the waist. In addition, axial skeletal pain (cervical spine or anterior chest or thoracic spine or low back) must be present. In this definition shoulder and buttock pain is considered as pain for each involved side. Low back pain is considered lower segment pain.
2. Pain in 11 of 18 tender point sites on digital palpation	Definition. Pain on digital palpation must be present in a least 11 of the following 18 tender point sites: Occiput: bilateral, at the suboccipital muscle insertion Low cervical: bilateral, at the anterior aspect of the intertransverse spaces at C5–C7 Trapezius: bilateral, at the midpoint of the upper border Supraspinatus: bilateral, at origins above the medial border of the scapular spine Second rib: bilateral, upper surfaces just lateral to the costochondral junctions Lateral epicondyle: bilateral, 2 cm distal to the epicondyles Gluteal: bilateral, in upper outer quadrants of buttocks in anterior fold of muscle Greater trochanter: bilateral, posterior to the trochanteric prominence Knee: bilateral, at the medial fat pad proximal to the joint line Digital palpation should be performed with a force of 4 kg. For a tender point to be considered 'positive' the subject must state that the palpation was painful; 'tender' is not to be considered 'painful'.

Note: For classification purposes, patients will be said to have fibromyalgia if both criteria are satisfied. Widespread pain must have been present for at least 3 months. The presence of a second clinical disorder does not exclude the diagnosis of fibromyalgia.

SLEEP DISTURBANCE

Patients have neither difficulty getting off to sleep nor problems with waking during the night, but they awake in the morning feeling tired and non-refreshed – so-called non-restorative sleep. The abnormality occurs in non-REM sleep. During normal non-REM sleep EEG recordings show δ waves at a frequency of 0.5–2 Hz. In FMS patients this pattern is interrupted by faster α waves at a frequency of 7.5–11 Hz. If non-REM sleep is disturbed in healthy volunteers, α intrusion is seen on the EEG and they describe symptoms of muscular fatigue and aching and the development of tender points. It is not clear whether these sleep disturbances may be the cause or the consequence of fibromyalgia pain.

PSYCHOLOGICAL INFLUENCES

Depression and anxiety disorders are commoner in patients with FMS than normal controls, but not necessarily in comparison with those with other pain syndromes. There is considerable overlap with allied conditions thought to have a psychological component, such as irritable bowel syndrome, chronic fatigue syndrome, dysmenorrhoea and premenstrual syndrome.

PATHOPHYSIOLOGY

The aetiology of FMS is unclear. A number of histological changes in the muscle of FMS patients have been described, including degenerative features and mitochondrial abnormalities. Tissue hypoxia, alteration in adenosine triphosphate (ATP) handling and abnormalities of muscle blood flow have all been described, but it is not known whether these findings are universal. Similarly, a number of neuropeptide changes have been noted, particularly depletion of serotonin and its precursor tryptophan. The role of substance P is unclear: elevated levels have been found in the CSF of FMS patients, but other studies have shown low or normal levels. The association with a number of autoimmune diseases has suggested that the immune system may be involved, but again findings are inconsistent.

MANAGEMENT

Although the diagnosis of FMS can be made with reasonable accuracy, the management is problematical. Only 5% of patients have complete remission of symptoms and the majority continue to have pain despite treatment. Therapy is summarized in Table 17.2.

TABLE 17.2 Management of fibromyalgia syndrome

Management	*Comments*
Medication	
Antidepressants	
Amitriptyline	Reasonable trials show improvement in some symptoms. Therapeutic effect may relate to effect on sleep – causes REM supression and prolongs non-REM sleep, thereby improving non-restorative sleep patterns
Dothiepin	Less literature available but may be useful
Fluoxetine	May be useful
Phenothiazines	May improve sleep disturbance but use limited by side-effects
NSAIDs and steroids	Probably no better than placebo
Injection therapy	
Regional sympathetic blockade, e.g. stellate ganglion block	May diminish tender points and pain. Probably works by increasing muscle blood flow or modulating hyperalgesia. Limited usefulness because pain is widespread
Tender point injections	May be injected with local anaesthetic +/– steroid. Patients have large numbers of tender points, so may be impractical
Fitness training	Rigorous (aerobic) cardiovascular fitness training may result in some objective and subjective improvement compared to flexibility exercises. May decrease the number of tender points
EMG biofeedback	Open trials suggest may reduce stiffness and number of tender points. May be mediated via ACTH and endorphins
Cognitive behavioural therapy	Multidisciplinary approach combines elements of exercise, biofeedback etc. with use of relaxation and cognitive techniques. Improves a number of psychological variables, including affective distress, sense of control and functional capacity

MYOFASCIAL PAIN SYNDROME

Myofascial pain syndrome (MPS) is a localized pain disorder. Patients usually complain of pain and tenderness in one quadrant of the body (or more localized, e.g. one muscle). Areas of localized tenderness are palpable lying in taut nodules or bands within the muscle. The localized tenderness is called a trigger point (TP) and is characteristic of MPS. Palpation of the TP typically elicits a zone of radiating pain or, less commonly, altered sensation. In addition, a local muscle twitch response may be elicited by snapping the taut muscle band. The twitch can be seen and also recorded electrically.

CLINICAL FEATURES

As with FMS the condition presents more commonly in females than males (3:1). Diagnostic criteria have been described for MPS (Table 17.3), although they lack the sensitivity and specificity of those for FMS.

TPs may be seen in normal subjects who are not complaining of pain. To make the diagnosis all five major criteria and at least one minor criterion must be satisfied.

TABLE 17.3 Diagnostic criteria for myofascial pain syndrome

Major criteria	*Minor criteria*
Regional pain complaint	Reproduction of clinical pain complaint or altered sensation by pain on the tender spot
Pain complaint or altered sensation in the distribution of referred pain from myofascial trigger point	Elicitation of a local twitch response by transverse snapping palpation of the tender spot or by needle insertion into the tender spot in the taut band
Taut band palpable in an accesible muscle	Pain alleviated by elongation (stretching) the muscle or by injecting the tender spot
Exquisite spot tenderness at one point along the length of the taut band	
Some degree of restricted range of motion when measurable	

PATHOPHYSIOLOGY

As with FMS, the underlying pathology is unclear. The key event is probably local muscle injury, which may be precipitated by trauma, overuse or abnormal posture. Local contracture then develops. Histological examination of TPs show changes similar to those of FMS.

MANAGEMENT

There are few good clinical studies of the treatment of MPS and many therapies are anecdotally based. The mainstays of management are inactivation of trigger points and avoidance of contributing factors. These treatments should be reinforced by exercise to minimize recurrence of the condition. As with other chronic painful conditions, psychological management plays an important role. Key management points are summarized in Table 17.4.

Treatment of MPS may take many years, although the prognosis is rather more favourable than for FMS.

TABLE 17.4 Treatment of myofascial pain syndrome

Management	*Comments*
Inactivation of trigger points	
Counterstimulation	Stretch and spray therapy well described: involves passive stretching of muscular TP while administering vapocoolant spray. May reduce TP tenderness and referred pain. Other techniques include TENS, massage, ultrasound and ice packs
Trigger point injection	Mechanical disruption of TP is more important than substance injected. Local anaesthetic injections are more comfortable than dry needling and may be co-administered with depot steroid preparations. Repeated injections may be necessary. Range of motion and exercise tolerance are increased. Acupuncture may also cause disruption of TP
Avoidance of contributing factors	Overuse of muscles, trauma, prolonged spasm and poor posture predispose to development of TPs. Precipitating factors in the workplace and at home can be identified and eliminated. Correction of mechanical abnormalities such as scoliosis and leg length discrepancy may improve symptoms
Psychological management	Psychological factors may be responsible for much of the morbidity. Multidisciplinary cognitive behavioural approach may produce best results in MPS

CHAPTER 18

SCAR PAIN

INTRODUCTION

Pain may persist in a surgical scar well after healing has taken place. Scars which commonly cause problems are those in the lower abdomen, such as following inguinal herniorrhaphy, Pfannenstiel incision for caesarian section or gynaecological procedures, or appendicectomy. Any operative or traumatic scar can cause persistent pain and treatment is similar whatever the site.

PATHOPHYSIOLOGY

Pain may be the result of a mechanical effect related to intermittent nerve or muscle compression, or local irritation from implanted foreign bodies. Re-exploration may be appropriate but this may cause further scarring. The condition more usually represents a form of neuropathic pain following 'nerve damage' at surgery. This leads to peripheral and central hyperexcitability, with associated phenomena such as hyperalgesia and allodynia. In addition (in common with other damaged primary afferents) enhanced sensitivity to sympathetic efferent activity may occur, manifesting as changes in skin colour and blood flow and abnormal temperature sensitivity adjacent to the scar.

CLINICAL FEATURES

Pain is sited adjacent to the scar or nearby, but may radiate widely. It is often stabbing or shooting in nature and is exacerbated by movement. Coughing, sneezing or straining may also worsen symptoms. Sensitivity to temperature may reflect associated autonomic dysfunction.

On examination the scar often looks well healed but there may be keloid formation. It may be tender to palpation along part or whole of its length. Careful palpation may reveal a neuroma. Adjacent areas of skin may exhibit hyper- or hypoalgesia, loss of sensation or allodynia.

MANAGEMENT

This is summarized in Table 18.1.

TABLE 18.1 Management of scar pain

Treatment	*Comments*
Injection therapy Local infiltration *Local anaesthetic +/– depot steroid*	Successive injections tend to provide longer-lasting relief. Little is to be gained from more than three injections
Neurolytic (6% aqueous phenol or absolute alcohol)	Useful if local anaesthetic blocks have given effective but transient relief. Results are often disappointing
Neurodestructive procedures (cryotherapy/RF lesioning)	Useful if local anaesthetic blocks have given effective but transient relief. Require accurate location of trigger point
Surgical exploration	Useful if a mechanical cause for pain is suspected
Pharmacotherapy Conventional analgesics *(NSAIDs/opioids)*	Usually ineffective
Amitriptyline	Probably best first-line drug
Anticonvulsants	May be helpful if lancinating component
TENS	Useful if no allodynia or hyperaesthesia
Psychological support	Often considerable psychological component, depending on significance of scar

CHAPTER 19

NEUROPATHIC PAIN

NEUROPATHIC PAIN

INTRODUCTION

Neuropathic pain is caused by a lesion or dysfunction in the nociceptive pathway. It may be divided into peripheral neuropathic pain and central pain, but many conditions have elements of both peripheral and central disturbance in sensory processing. Many conditions may result in nervous system damage, including trauma or surgery, chemotherapy, radiotherapy, vascular insult, infection, diabetes, AIDS or malignancy. A number of chronic pain syndromes which are not related to obvious nerve injury appear to have a neuropathic component.

CLINICAL FEATURES

Whatever the nature of nervous tissue dysfunction, a number of characteristic symptoms are described in pain of neuropathic origin:

- **Spontaneous pain** (in the absence of obvious peripheral stimulus), which may be paroxysmal or continuous. The pain is described as arising in skin (burning, pricking, stabbing), muscle or bone (aching, cramping, throbbing). Electric shock-type shooting pain is frequently reported.
- **Allodynia** – pain following an innocuous stimulus.
- **Hyperalgesia** – pain of abnormal severity following a noxious stimulus.
- **Hyperpathia** – increased pain in an area of increased sensory threshold (the pain may follow noxious or innocuous stimuli).

PATHOPHYSIOLOGY

Nerve damage results in a number of peripheral and central effects.

PERIPHERAL SEQUELAE OF NERVE DAMAGE

- Sensitization of peripheral nociceptors, including reduced threshold for activation and enhanced response to suprathreshold stimuli
- Ectopic impulse generation, which occurs in both Aδ and C fibres and in dorsal root ganglia. Spontaneous electrical activity can be demonstrated in neuromata following nerve transection. Microneuromata may result from incomplete nerve injury, e.g. in postherpetic neuralgia. The effect is probably mediated through sodium channel accumulation in damaged afferents
- Abnormal sensitivity to sympathetic efferent activity (see Chapter 1).

CENTRAL SEQUELAE OF (PERIPHERAL) NERVE DAMAGE

- Sensitization of spinal cord neurones by afferent C-fibre nociceptive activity. C-fibre input activates glutaminergic synapses of the *N*-methyl-D-aspartate (NMDA) type. A number of postsynaptic sequelae give rise to enhanced nociceptive transmission despite diminished peripheral input
- Altered supraspinal control of afferent input to the cord is likely to occur with changing afferent input following nerve damage
- Trophic and metabolic influences induce changes in the central nervous system, including downregulation and upregulation of peptides involved in nociceptive processing and reduction in nerve growth factor and other substances involved in normal sensory processing.

Remember: Many of the clinical features of neuropathic pain are the result of CNS changes induced by peripheral events. Primary damage to nociceptive pathways in the CNS produces a similar clinical picture (allodynia, hyperpathia, spontaneous pain etc.) to that following peripheral injury. There is often a delay (up to years) between the central injury and the onset of pain symptoms.

TREATMENT

Neuropathic pain is notoriously refractory to treatment. The mainstays of therapy are pharmacological, but no treatment is universally successful. The most commonly used classes of drugs are the tricyclic antidepressants, membrane-stabilizing agents and topical preparations. There is rationale for the use of other classes of drugs, such as the NMDA channel blockers. The role of opioids in the management of neuropathic pain remains controversial. These classes of drugs have been fully discussed in Chapters 2–7, but a brief overview of their use in the management of neuropathic pain will be given to underpin descriptions of specific neuropathic pain states.

TRICYCLIC ANTIDEPRESSANTS

The use of tricyclic antidepressants in the management of neuropathic pain is supported by large numbers of controlled trials. The best-studied and most commonly used drugs are the first-generation drugs, including amitriptyline, doxepin desipramine, clomipramine and dothiepin. It is now clear that these relieve pains with a number of different characteristics (i.e. burning, shooting, aching, stabbing), and both continuous and paroxysmal pains. Studies excluding depressed patients and including only depressed patients, and in which mood was carefully evaluated, confirm that the analgesic effects of these drugs are separate from their mood-altering actions.

These drugs block reuptake of CNS monoamines, particularly noradrenaline and serotonin, in addition to a number of other neurotransmitters. They may alter nociceptive processing in the CNS by prolonging the synaptic activity of these amines, thereby enhancing inhibitory (descending) nociceptive pathways. Amitriptyline and imipramine are mixed reuptake blockers (noradrenaline and serotonin). Side-effects (which may limit their use) are sedative and anticholinergic, particularly dry mouth. Urinary retention and constipation are less common but well documented problems. In an attempt to reduce these side-effects the relatively selective noradrenergic blockers such as desipramine have been used, with good results. Selective serotonergic blockers such as fluoxetine do not appear to relieve pain when used alone, but in mixed uptake blockers the serotonergic effect possibly enhances the noradrenergic effect.

The starting dose of these drugs should be small, e.g. amitriptyline 10 mg or 25 mg, and increased incrementally every 5–7 days. It is suggested that the drug be taken at night to minimize daytime drowsiness (the sedative effect may be beneficial for those whose sleep is disturbed by pain). If morning drowsiness does occur patients should be advised that they will become tolerant to this effect over a short period. Although some analgesic benefit may be noticed within a week it its worth pointing out that the medication may have to be taken for several weeks before an improvement in symptoms is seen. The effective dose varies between patients, and there are a few good studies relating serum concentrations to efficacy.

MEMBRANE-STABILIZING DRUGS

These drugs are known to suppress ectopic impulse generation in damaged nervous tissue by their sodium channel blocking effects. The doses required to block abnormal impulse generation are considerably lower than those required to suppress normal electrical activity.

Anticonvulsants

The use of carbamazepine in trigeminal neuralgia is well established. This and other anticonvulsants, such as sodium valproate, phenytoin and clonazepam, may modify the experience of neuropathic pain. Previously used only for shooting, electric shock-type pains, it is now known that they can modify other abnormal sensory phenomena.

Local anaesthetic drugs

Lignocaine by intravenous infusion may relieve pain in a number of neuropathic conditions. Concentrations are much lower than those needed for axonal blockade. Its use is predominantly diagnostic, predicting likely response to oral membrane stabilizers. Unfortunately, some patients who have complete pain relief with intravenous lignocaine do not achieve similar symptomatic relief from subsequent therapy with anticonvulsants/antiarrhythmics.

Antiarrythmic drugs

Mexiletine and tocainide block voltage-dependent sodium channels. The use of these drugs should be carefully supervised because of cardiovascular side-effects. Good efficacy data are not yet available.

TOPICAL THERAPY

Most of the work on topical therapy has been related to the study of postherpetic neuralgia, although other conditions in which allodynia is prominent may benefit from topical treatment.

Capsaicin preparations

Capsaicin is a natural product extracted from chilli peppers. It stimulates the release of substance P from primary afferent C-fibre terminals. On first application this causes a burning sensation which diminishes with repeated application as depletion of substance P occurs. Capsaicin may deplete substance P and other neuropeptides centrally. Capsaicin extract is available commercially in the UK as a 0.075% preparation. The analgesic effect may take several days to appear and patients should be advised that the initial burning on application should resolve with repeated use.

Topical NSAIDs

A number of topical NSAIDs have been used in the treatment of postherpetic neuralgia, with varying reports of success. These include topical benzydamine, aspirin in chloroform, and the application of indomethacin as an adherent medicated cloth. These agents are thought to work by local cyclo-oxygenase inhibition in the region of cutaneous nociceptors. Additional effects may include local membrane stabilization and blockade of receptors of inflammatory mediators. The promising reports of efficacy of these treatments need to be substantiated by well conducted controlled trials.

Topical local anaesthetic drugs

Damaged peripheral nerves are susceptible to the (sodium channel blocking) effects of local anaesthetics, and the development of topically acting preparations of lignocaine/prilocaine and amethocaine holds promise for the treatment of conditions such as postherpetic neuralgia. Further data relating to their long-term use are needed.

OPIOIDS AND NEUROPATHIC PAIN

Traditional teaching suggested that neuropathic pain was unresponsive to opioids. Mechanisms of opioid resistance include downregulation of opioid receptors in response to injurious stimuli, elaboration of antalgesic peptides and degeneration of inhibitory interneurones. More recent work using unrestricted patient-controlled analgesia systems suggest that with sufficient dosage many neuropathic pains may be opioid responsive. Such findings suggest that opioid therapy should be evaluated in patients whose pain has not responded to other treatments.

DRUGS INFLUENCING NMDA RECEPTOR ACTIVITY

Afferent C-fibre nociceptive activity leads to the release of the excitatory neurotransmitters glutamate and aspartate which, via their action at *N*-methyl-D-aspartate-type receptors, lead to central hyperexcitability. NMDA antagonism would therefore be expected to be a useful analgesic tool. Although glutamate release inhibitors such as lamotrigine are of theoretical benefit, clinical experience is disappointing. The most readily available NMDA antagonist for clinical use is the phencyclidine derivative ketamine. Several studies have now demonstrated its efficacy in a number of neuropathic pain states, including postherpetic neuralgia. Its clinical use is limited by sedative and psychomimetic side-effects. Long-term administration may be difficult as reliable dosing cannot be achieved with oral administration, and there are few safety data relating to its extended use.

PHANTOM LIMB PAIN

INTRODUCTION

This is classically described as pain referred to a surgically removed limb or portion thereof, but it is also seen following accidental amputation. Phantom pains have also been described following mastectomy, removal of teeth, gastrectomy and excision of genitalia. A closely related phenomenon is that of deafferentation pain, such as occurs following brachial plexus avulsion or spinal cord injury. Stump pain may occur in isolation without associated phantom experiences, and is usually due to neuroma formation (see below).

AETIOLOGY

The cause of the pain is uncertain but probably results from interaction between peripheral and central mechanisms. It is possible that different factors predominate in different patients, which would account for the inconsistent responses to therapy. Possible anatomical origins of the pain include:

- **the amputation stump** – regenerating axon sprouts from cut peripheral nerves form neuromata, in which spontaneous electrical activity has been demonstrated. Sensitive neuromata are frequently palpable in amputation stumps. Abolition of afferent input from these neuromata, either pharmacologically or with cryotherapy or radiofrequency destruction, may be helpful in the treatment of phantom limb pain.
- **the spinal cord** – when peripheral nerves are cut, changes in their central terminations may be noted. These include depletion of neurochemicals, facilitation of synaptic transmission and alteration in receptive fields of dorsal horn neurones. Likely to be involved in perpetuation of pain despite diminished/absent afferent input.
- **the brain** – phantom limb pain is such a complex sensory experience that it is likely to be integrated in the brain. Plastic changes in the brain occur in response to injury. It has been suggested that a pain 'memory' or engram is established prior to amputation, hence the similarities seen between the pain and preamputation experience.

CLINICAL FEATURES

Almost all amputees experience some type of phantom sensation. Painless phenomena are common and range from ill-defined sensations in the missing limb to a complete awareness of the limb, including size, posture movement and temperature. The incidence of pain in the phantom limb is probably as high as 60% in the months following amputation, and persisting pain occurs in about 10% of patients, i.e. the incidence decreases with time. Prolonged pain prior to amputation appears to be associated with an increased incidence of the condition, whereas age and reason for amputation are less important. Pain is typically described as gripping, crushing or tearing, and most often occurs in the hand or foot of the amputated limb. The pain is often qualitatively similar to that experienced prior to amputation. 'Telescoping' of the limb (where the position of the amputated hand or foot approaches the stump) appears to correlate with a reduction in symptoms and an improved prognosis. Unpleasant emotional experiences exacerbate the pain.

MANAGEMENT

PREVENTION

Phantom limb pain seems to be related to modification of the nervous system in response to the pain of a diseased limb, and also to the barrage of nociceptive information at the time of amputation. Provision of analgesia, preferably by axonal blockade prior to and at the time of amputation, seems to reduce the incidence of the condition. Similarly, if effective pain relief is instituted early in the course of the disease the outcome is likely to be more favourable.

OTHER TREATMENTS

Such pain is notoriously difficult to treat: at least 70 treatments have been described, none of which is even moderately successful. The most commonly used are outlined in Table 19.1. As with many chronic pain conditions, a combination of therapies may be successful.

TABLE 19.1 Management of phantom limb pain

Treatment	*Comments*
Physical techniques	
Excision of neuroma/refashioning of stump	Further neuromata formation likely
Cryotherapy/radiofrequency lesioning	More useful in stump than in phantom pain
Cordotomy	Requires considerable skill, may produce further pain
Dorsal root entry zone lesion	Rarely successful
Local anaesthetic techniques	
Stump infiltration	Rarely successful as sole technique; also short-lived effect
Epidural analgesia	Quite useful in short term but requires long-term spinal drug delivery system to be useful as definitive treatment
Modification of autonomic nervous system	
Lumbar sympathectomy/stellate ganglion block	Useful in some cases
Conventional analgesics	
Non-steroidal anti-inflammatory drugs	Clinically seem to be ineffective, but central actions of drugs may make them useful adjuncts to other therapy
Opioids	Nerve injury often reduces sensitivity to opioids
Other drugs	
Anticonvulsants, e.g. Sodium valproate and tricyclic antidepressants, e.g. amitriptyline	Useful first-line therapy for neuropathic pain. Anticonvulsants said to be particularly useful for shooting/lancinating pain but not exclusively so
NMDA channel blockers, e.g. ketamine	Useful in some patients but more trials needed
Stimulation techniques	
TENS	Simple, safe, and may augment other therapies
Dorsal column stimulation	Useful in some cases
Deep brain stimulation	Little evidence for efficacy
Acupuncture	Efficacy not supported by controlled trials but reported to be useful
Behavioural therapy	May be valuable adjunct to other treatments

POSTHERPETIC NEURALGIA

DEFINITION

Postherpetic neuralgia (PHN) is a common cause of neuropathic pain. It is the most common and feared complication of herpes zoster infection. PHN occurs when there is continuing pain beyond the normal time of healing of the rash (and should be distinguished from acute herpetic neuralgia, which refers to pain experienced before and in the presence of the characteristic skin lesions). The pain tends to resolve with time (only 10–25% of those with PHN after 1 month still have pain at a year), and PHN has been variously defined as pain persisting beyond 1 and 6 months after the appearance of the rash. It should probably be defined as pain persisting for more than 3 months after the acute period (or 4 months from the appearance of the rash).

INCIDENCE

The incidence of the condition is variably reported as occurring in 10–75% of patients with herpes zoster infection. The true incidence depends on the definition used and is markedly influenced by the age of the patient, the condition being much more common in elderly patients. Furthermore, this incidence may represent a wide clinical spectrum, ranging from mild short-lived discomfort to prolonged intractable severe pain. The lack of a universally accepted definition and the tendency for symptoms to resolve spontaneously make it difficult to assess risk factors for PHN and to compare treatments for the condition.

PATHOPHYSIOLOGY

ACUTE HERPES ZOSTER

Varicella zoster virus infection manifests initially as chickenpox, usually in children. In immunocompetent children it is usually a mild disease with little morbidity. Primary varicella in adults tends to be a more serious condition. Following resolution of the initial infection the virus persists in latent form in dorsal root ganglia. Many years later the virus is reactivated and causes herpes zoster. It is not known what causes reactivation of the virus but it may be infection, immunosuppression or malignancy. Usually there is no precipitating cause. The virus replicates in the dorsal root ganglion and is transported distally along sensory nerves, producing the characteristic dermatomal rash of shingles. Pain may occur a few days before appearance of the rash (preherpetic neuralgia) and continues until skin lesions disappear.

It can be dull, sharp, aching or shooting. Paraesthesia and hyperaesthesia are common during the acute stage. The rash is at first papular, progressing to a vesicular then pustular stage, after which crusting occurs. The crusting usually disappears after 4–5 weeks, leaving scarring. Pain and sensory disturbances usually resolve at this time.

The lesions appear most commonly in thoracic dermatomes and are usually unilateral. The second most common site is the ophthalmic division of the trigeminal nerve, particularly in the elderly (this may lead to corneal scarring). A single dorsal root ganglion or a small number of adjacent ones may be affected, and they appear haemorrhagic and swollen on microscopy. Degeneration in posterior nerve roots is seen. Very occasionally the anterior horn may be involved, resulting in motor paralysis in the affected area.

POSTHERPETIC NEURALGIA

Pathological studies in patients with postherpetic neuralgia have shown a number of changes in nervous tissue, but these have also been seen in patients without persisting pain. Findings include dorsal horn atrophy, axonal and myelin loss, and fibrosis in dorsal root ganglia. There is a relative reduction in the large myelinated fibre population, with preservation of small myelinated and unmyelinated fibres. Normal modulation of small fibre activity by large fibre input is lost, which may partly explain why pain persists.

CLINICAL FEATURES

The diagnosis of PHN is usually easy because there is a history of shingles. The pain experienced in the acute phase persists. It is typically continuous and is described as burning or aching, with characteristic shooting or stabbing exacerbations. The pain is accompanied by hyperaesthesia and allodynia, although the scars themselves may be hypoaesthetic. Itching is often a prominent feature. Occasionally patients present with this typical pain when the skin manifestations have completely disappeared.

MANAGEMENT

PREVENTION

It has been postulated that early resolution of the acute herpes zoster illness will reduce the incidence of PHN. This has not been repeatedly substantiated, although prompt management may enhance the efficacy of subsequent treatment. As with treatment of established PHN, the high spontaneous resolution rate makes it difficult to evaluate prophylactic measures. Prophylactic treatments are summarized in Table 19.2.

TABLE 19.2 Management of postherpetic neuralgia: prophylactic measures

Treatment	*Comments*
Topical idoxuridine in DMSO (dimethyl sulphoxide)	Promotes early healing of vesicles and reduction in pain. Small studies show reduced incidence of PHN, but not confirmed in larger groups
Systemic antiviral agents (Acyclovir/famcyclovir)	Proven benefit in acute stage, but existing evidence neither confirms nor refutes that these (expensive) treatments reduce incidence and severity of PHN. Antivirals may change quality of postherpetic pain
Systemic corticosteroids	May provide short-term relief in acute phase, but side-effects of longer-term use limit utility in preventing PHN
Nerve blocks	
Infiltration	Uncontrolled reports that subcutaneous infiltration with 0.2% triamcinolone in saline reduces symptoms in acute stage and may reduce incidence of PHN
Somatic	May provide temporary symptomatic relief but probably do not reduce incidence of PHN
Autonomic	Sympathetic blockade may provide immediate pain relief and early healing of vesicles. If instituted early *may* reduce incidence of PHN
Vaccination	Still developmental – effect on acute herpes zoster and PHN unknown

TREATMENT OF POSTHERPETIC NEURALGIA

Many treatments for this condition are described in the literature: many are anecdotal and the results of well controlled trials are often contradictory. Currently the mainstays of treatment are adrenergically/serotonergically active antidepressants, such as **amitriptyline** and topical **capsaicin**. The rationale for their use, suggested doses and side-effects are discussed in Chapter 6. These and other treatments are summarized in Table 19.3.

Postherpetic neuralgia is a debilitating condition and patients will be helped by the usual psychological interventions available in the pain clinic.

CONCLUSION

The natural course of PHN is one of improvement, and patients should be reassured on this point. The role of preventive measures in the acute stage remains speculative. Successful treatment outcomes are much more likely when the interval between the acute infection and initiation of treatment is short, therefore early and appropriate treatment is desirable in patients suffering from PHN.

TABLE 19.3 Management of postherpetic neuralgia

Treatment	*Comments*
Drug therapy	
Tricyclic antidepressants	Several controlled studies suggest amitriptyline beneficial in PHN. Useful first-line therapy. Seems to be more effective the earlier it is started. Other tricyclics and other classes of antidepressants seem less successful
Anticonvulsants *(Carbemazepine/sodium valproate)*	Probably less successful than antidepressants, with which they are often co-prescribed. Especially helpful in patients with shooting/electric shock-type sensations
Antiarrythmics	
Mexiletine	May reduce ectopic impulse generation from damaged primary afferents. Useful response to intravenous lignocaine may predict success of this drug.
Ketamine	Probably works via NMDA blockade.
Opioid analgesics	Role remains controversial. i.v. opioids certainly control pain in some patients. Sustained-release preparations useful for long-term therapy.
Topical therapy	
Capsaicin 0.075% cream	Useful first-line treatment in PHN (despite expense). Well conducted trials support its use
Topical NSAIDs	Indomethacin or aspirin reported to be more effective than benzydamine
Aspirin 0.4% in chloroform	Open studies describe excellent results. Cheap and easy to make up. Appears to work better than chloroform alone. Needs repeated application (usually t.d.s.) for long-term pain control
Topical local anaesthetic *EMLA/lignocaine gel 5–10%*	Provide short-term relief when applied but not clear whether useful for long-term therapy
Nerve blocks	Both somatic and autonomic blocks may provide transient relief in PHN, but probably not useful for long-term management
Other treatments	
Neurostimulation techniques	
TENS	Rarely alleviates pain completely but may give some improvement. Most of the evidence for its use is anecdotal
DCS/DBS	Uncommon for DCS to provide sustained relief. Thalamic stimulation may be beneficial in some patients. Invasive techniques should only be considered when other measures have failed
Acupuncture	Poor results in PHN
Surgery	Destructive techniques have poor success and may themselves cause neuropathic pain. Dorsal root entry zone (DREZ) lesioning seems to be the most successful of these techniques.

CENTRAL POST-STROKE PAIN

INTRODUCTION

Central post-stroke pain (CPSP) is a neuropathic pain syndrome following a stroke. It is characterized by pain and sensory loss in the body part that corresponds with the whole or part of the cerebrovascular lesion. It was originally termed thalamic pain, but subsequent studies have shown that many lesions are extrathalamic. The condition occurs in about 8% of stroke patients and probably affects more than 6000 patients per year in the UK.

CLINICAL FEATURES

Just over half of patients will develop pain within 1 month of the stroke, but the appearance of symptoms may be delayed for as long as 34 months. Motor impairment is often mild in cases of CPSP. Pain is often experienced in a large part of the left or right side. The pain is typically described as burning, but shooting/lancinating pains are also common. Patients will often describe the pain as severe and comment that it is exacerbated by cold or emotional stress. Body movement may exacerbate the pain.

Examination reveals typical findings:

- There is almost always a sensory deficit, with over 99% of patients showing decreased sensation to pinprick and heat (warm and cold).
- The area of sensory change is usually greater than the area in which pain is described.
- Abnormal evoked sensations are common.
- Over half of patients have demonstrable touch and cold allodynia, and a greater proportion show dysaesthesia to touch and cold. The allodynic area tends to correspond with that in which the pain occurs.
  NB: Abnormal evoked sensations are rare in stroke patients without pain.

PATHOPHYSIOLOGY

The condition appears to be the result of a lesion in the spinothalamocortical pathway, although not all patients with such a lesion will experience pain. It appears to be characterized by hyperexcitability of the thalamic or cortical neurones, which have lost their usual input.

TREATMENT

The general principles of management of neuropathic pain apply. Typically the pain is resistant to conventional treatment, including opioids. Therapeutic options are summarized in Table 19.4.

TABLE 19.4 Management of central post-stroke pain

Treatment	*Comments*
Antidepressants	Should probably be used as first-line drugs. Their efficacy may correspond with plasma levels, but plasma level does not correspond with dose! Adrenergically active drugs, e.g. amitriptyline, seem most effective
Anticonvulsants	Not useful as sole therapy but may be useful adjunct to tricyclic antidepressants. One good controlled trial suggests that carbamazepine may not be useful, so sodium valproate probably best first-line anticonvulsant. **NB**: Vigabatrin (GABA agonist) may be helpful for allodynia
Antiarrhythmics	Controlled trials suggest that intravenous lignocaine may have short-term benefit. Oral mexiletine may provide longer-term relief
Naloxone	Used to be the recommended treatment for CPSP. Has been given in large doses (up to 50 mg) but 12 mg is a more usual dose. Said to give long-lasting relief in many patients. Previously suggested that it increased perfusion to injured brain – others suggested that it increased levels of endogenous opioids. Double-blind randomized controlled trials appear to show no benefit
Opioids	Not sensible first-line drugs but some patients may respond. Response should be assessed carefully in each individual before prescribing long-term therapy
Neurostimulation	
TENS	Useful for patients who have intact touch/vibration sense
Brain stimulation	Chronic motor cortex stimulation, described as successful, although effect not well sustained. Stimulation needs to be carried out in the area of cortex that controls motor function in the painful part
Spinal cord stimulation	May be useful if pain is felt in a limb

CONCLUSION

CPSP is not uncommon and therefore those looking after stroke patients should ask about symptoms of pain. If a diagnosis is made, early appropriate treatment should be started. **If unsuccessful, pain clinic help should be sought**.

COMPLEX REGIONAL PAIN SYNDROME

INTRODUCTION

There are a number of painful conditions where the symptom pattern suggests involvement of the sympathetic nervous system in the underlying pathophysiology. Such conditions can often be relieved by blockade of (efferent) sympathetic activity to the painful area. Many neuropathic conditions will partially benefit from sympathetic blockade, and such pains may be said to be *sympathetically maintained*. However, a more specific group of conditions are typified by sensory, autonomic and motor symptoms but clinical features and response to sympathetic blockade are inconsistent, which has hampered satisfactory classification. This led in 1995 to a revised taxonomy of these conditions, which are now categorized as complex regional pain syndromes (CRPS). They are so called because they have varied clinical manifestations (i.e. *complex*) and they usually affect the distal part of a limb (i.e. *regional*).

There are two categories:

- **CRPS type I** (formerly known as reflex sympathetic dystrophy) – This develops after a noxious inciting event (major or trivial), which may be local or distant (e.g. stroke, myocardial infarction).
- **CRPS type II** (formerly causalgia) – This develops following a nerve injury (often median or sciatic).

NB: In both groups the symptoms and signs are disproportionate to the magnitude of the inciting event.

The clinical phenomenology and underlying pathophysiology of the two groups are similar and will be discussed together.

CLINICAL FEATURES

(**NB**: not all patients will have all symptoms!)

SITE

CRPS usually affects one extremity, more commonly an upper limb. Less commonly the condition is bilateral. The distal part of the limb is affected in a generalized manner, i.e. not in the distribution of a single peripheral nerve (or particularly of the injured nerve in CRPS type II). However, the condition can also affect other sites, such as the side of the face or the trunk.

PAIN

Pain tends to be throbbing, burning or shooting, and is usually felt to be 'deep' within the affected extremity. It is usually exacerbated when the limb is dependent or is moved. Local or environmental temperature changes also tend to exacerbate symptoms. In addition, evoked pain, i.e. hyperalgesia and allodynia, are common.

AUTONOMIC DYSFUNCTION

This is suggested by:

- **Skin blood flow abnormality** – The affected extremity will often be discoloured (red, blue, mottled) and is often hotter or colder than the non-affected limb.
- **Abnormalities of sweating** – May be hyper or hypohydrotic.
- **Oedema** – Commonly present particularly on the dorsum of the hand or foot. The overlying skin is often shiny.

There are a number of other characteristics seen in CRPS but which are **not necessary for the diagnosis**.

- **Motor dysfunction** – This occurs late in the condition and is seen frequently. Features include weakness or paresis, limited active range of movement, tremor (postural or action) and dystonia (rare).
- **Trophic changes** – These also tend to occur late in the condition, and include disturbed nail/hair growth, hyperkeratosis, palmar/plantar fibrosis and distal osteoporosis. These features may be related to the underlying motor disturbance, i.e. the interaction between the two sets of features is complex.

> **Remember**: Combinations of symptoms vary between patients, and in a given patient at different times.

PATHOPHYSIOLOGY OF PAIN ASSOCIATED WITH AUTONOMIC DYSFUNCTION

The observation that CRPS may be relieved by sympathetic blockade suggests that the sympathetic nervous system is involved in the generation of pain. In addition, these painful conditions may be exacerbated by electrical stimulation of the sympathetic efferent pathways.

It now seems unlikely that these conditions result from excess sympathetic efferent activity, but rather from an abnormal response of the primary afferents to sympathetic stimulation. The following events may occur.

The initial inciting (noxious) event causes peripheral and central sensitization (see Chapter 1), with altered signal processing in the spinal cord. This is manifested by reduced excitatory thresholds of damaged afferents and ectopic impulse generation (probably brought about by alterations in the expression and disposition of sodium channels). Centrally there is facilitated transmission of nociceptive information.

In addition, traumatized afferents develop adrenoceptor sensitivity at their sensory endings, axonally and in the dorsal root ganglion, possibly as a result of upregulation or enhanced adrenoceptor expression in response to injury. This would provide a mechanism for chemical sympathetic/sensory coupling, whereby noradrenaline from sympathetic nerve endings acts on damaged afferents to produce further sensitization and impulse generation. Released noradrenaline may also act on presynaptic α-adrenoceptors, triggering the release of inflammatory mediators and enhancement of pain. The skin colour and temperature changes, as well as the oedema, may result from trauma-induced vascular smooth muscle sensitivity to noradrenaline.

The peripheral and central sensitization gives rise to the spontaneous pain, allodynia and hyperalgesia typical of these conditions.

MANAGEMENT

The mainstay of treatment of these conditions has been blockade of sympathetic efferent activity. Systemic administration of the α-adrenoceptor antagonist phentolamine (5–15 mg over 10 minutes) has been used as a diagnostic and therapeutically prognostic tool. Good response to intravenous phentolamine suggests that sympathetic block will produce pain relief.

Treatments are summarized in Table 19.5.

CONCLUSION

There are likely to be other pathophysiological mechanisms in the genesis of these pain states, and the natural progression of the disease is unknown. The mechanisms by which the sympathetic nervous system influences pain are complex but becoming increasingly understood. It seems that its role is to accentuate the post-injury phenomena seen in other neuropathic pain states. Treatment is currently based on anecdotal experience rather than evidence supported by double-blind randomized controlled trials, but given the likely pathophysiology, early mobilization and the use of drugs which ameliorate the sequelae of nerve injury would seem logical.

TABLE 19.5 Management of complex regional pain syndrome

Treatment	*Comments*
Intravenous regional sympathectomy *Procedure* Guanethidine 20 mg (upper limb) or 30 mg (lower limb) in saline or prilocaine. 20–30 ml are injected into the affected extremity distal to a suprasystolic tourniquet, which remains inflated for 20 minutes. Blocks may be performed repeatedly. **NB**: Reserpine, bretylium, ketanserin and NSAIDs have been used	This is currently the mainstay of treatment, although systematic review has cast doubt on its efficacy – guanethidine may be no better than placebo. The effect may be mediated by exsanguination or tourniquet. The technique is still in common use
Paravertebral sympatholysis Stellate ganglion block (for upper limb pain) *Procedure* Local anaesthetic, e.g. bupivacaine 0.5%. 5–10 ml are applied to the cervicothoracic ganglion in the neck. The procedure may be performed repeatedly.	Horner's syndrome suggests correct needle placement but a greater volume may be needed to block sympathetic efferents in the arm. Complications include laryngeal nerve block, blurred vision, intravascular injection, injection into CSF
Lumbar sympathetic block (for lower limb pain) *Procedure* Local anaesthetic, e.g. bupivacaine 0.25% or lignocaine 1% 10 ml or neurolytic, e.g. aqueous phenol 6%, alcohol 50% 5–7 ml are injected via a paravertebral needle at the level of L2/L3 to the lumbar sympathetic chain which lies along the anterolateral margins of the lumbar vertebrae	Complications include transient hypotension (suggests successful sympatholysis), somatic nerve damage and intravascular injection **NB**: Bilateral blocks may cause impotence.
Local anaesthetic blocks e.g. intrathecal, epidural, plexus blocks or peripheral nerve blocks	Block sympathetic fibres accompanying somatic nerves

TABLE 19.5 *(cont'd)*

Pharmacotherapy Amitriptyline Carbamazepine Sodium valproate Mexiletine NMDA channel blockers (may prevent central sensitization)	See under introduction to Neuropathic pain
Neurostimulation TENS	May be uncomfortable in presence of hyperalgesia/allodynia
Spinal cord stimulation	Alters autonomic responses in affected limb
Acupuncture	May be no better than sham acupuncture
Physiotherapy	Important not only in preventing the sequelae of the disease but as therapy per se. Other treatments, e.g. intravenous regional sympathectomy, should be performed in conjunction with physiotherapy, i.e. **physiotherapy should underpin all other treatments**

CHAPTER 20

FACIAL PAIN

TRIGEMINAL NEURALGIA

DEFINITION/INCIDENCE

Trigeminal neuralgia (TGN) is a severe paroxysmal facial pain which has a number of typical characteristics (see below). The condition may be severely disabling and morbidity, particularly in the elderly, may be high.

CLINICAL FEATURES

TGN is commonest in the 50–70-year age group. The diagnosis is based on the very typical history of the pain:

- **Site** – Almost exclusively in the distribution of the trigeminal nerve. Occurs in mandibular (3rd) division > maxillary (2nd) division > ophthalmic (1st) division. Combination of 3rd and 2nd divisions possibly most common. 3% of cases are bilateral, although symptoms tend to be unilateral during an attack. Pain may spread to a wider area with time. Some debate as to whether right-sided pain is commoner than that on the left.
- **Character** – The pain is described as stabbing, lancinating or electric shock-like, lasting for a few seconds. Onset and offset are abrupt.
- **Temporal nature** – The pain is paroxysmal in nature, with typical episodes lasting weeks or months followed by quiescent periods when the patient may be pain free for as long as several years. The frequency of attacks tends to increase with age.
- **Precipitating features** – The pain is almost always triggered by a non-noxious stimulus, usually in the nasolabial fold or perioral region. Washing, tooth cleaning, shaving, chewing, swallowing or talking are common precipitators. Exposure to cold may also trigger the pain. The trigger site may not be related to the distribution of the pain and activities such as hair brushing, which stimulate upper cervical segments, may result in trigeminal pain, although the trigger site is always ipsilateral to the pain.

EXAMINATION/SPECIAL INVESTIGATIONS

Because of the sensitivity of the trigger sites the patient with severe untreated TGN may present with poor oral hygiene, drooling at the mouth and emaciation due to poor food intake. They may be unshaven and unkempt; however, most patients will have brought their symptoms to the attention of a doctor at an earlier stage. The diagnosis is made on the history, but neurological examination reveals minimal or absent sensory changes in the distribution of the trigeminal nerve. Further investigations are rarely necessary, but MRI may show abnormal vasculature (see below) or other (rare) causative intracranial pathology.

PATHOPHYSIOLOGY

The condition is usually idiopathic but may be secondary to disseminated sclerosis, lesions in the cerebellopontine angle, or Vth nerve tumours, e.g. neuroma. Some patients give a history of trauma. Examination of nerve tissue from patients with TGN often shows local hypo- demyelination in the region of the trigeminal ganglion. The condition has clinical similarity to focal epilepsy, which suggests disturbances in the trigeminal root entry zone that generate repetitive action potentials. Neurosurgeons have observed that over 85% of patients have compression of the trigeminal root adjacent to the pons, usually by an artery. This has been confirmed by both autopsy studies and MRI findings. It is unclear why the trigger zone may be remote from the site of pain, but may be related to altered central connectivity.

MANAGEMENT (MEDICAL/SURGICAL)

The initial therapy of trigeminal neuralgia is pharmacological, with anticonvulsants. Carbamazepine is the mainstay of treatment. Local infiltration and nerve blocks may provide temporary relief. Neurodestructive procedures and craniotomy for microvascular decompression should be reserved for those who are unresponsive to or intolerant of medical therapy. Treatment options are summarized in Table 20.1.

MICROVASCULAR DECOMPRESSION

Suboccipital microvascular decompression gives long-term pain relief in 80–90% of cases of TGN. There must be no medical contraindication to craniotomy. Preoperative high-definition magnetic resonance tomographic angiography is a sensitive and specific method for demonstrating vascular compression in TGN, and allows appropriate selection of surgical cases. There are many retrospective follow-up series in the literature which suggest that the procedure has a mortality rate of 0.5%. Permanent cranial nerve complications occur in 5–10% of patients. There is a need for controlled prospective neurosurgical studies with independent assessments of outcome.

CONCLUSION

Untreated TGN can be severely disabling. The diagnosis is usually straightforward on the basis of the history. Because the pathophysiology of the condition is poorly understood the ideal therapy for the condition is unclear, although symptomatic relief may be achieved pharmacologically and surgical techniques appear to abolish symptoms in many cases.

TABLE 20.1 Management of trigeminal neuralgia

Treatment	*Comments*
Pharmacological	
Anticonvulsants	
Carbamazepine (CBZ)	Most commonly used first-line drug, with response rates reported between 50 and 90%. Side-effects occur in 20% of patients (see p. 97). Interactions see p. 98
Phenytoin	May be used as an adjunct to CBZ or when patient is intolerant or unresponsive to CBZ. Side-effects and drug interactions are common (see p. 98)
Sodium valproate	May be useful – often co-prescribed with tricyclic antidepressants
Clonazepam	Efficacy very variably reported. Use often limited by sedation
Other drugs	
Baclofen	Possibly synergistic with CBZ. Few published data about its sole use
Injection therapy	
Trigger point infiltration	Usually provides analgesia for the duration of the local anaesthetic, but analgesia for longer periods reported
Peripheral blockade	
Local anaesthetic	Provides analgesia for duration of local anaesthetic. Useful for allowing patients to experience areas of anaesthesia before permanent blockade
Phenol	Painful on injection. Sensory loss invariable and recurrence of pain occurs in 6–12 months.
Peripheral cryotherapy	Results in transient sensory loss. May be repeated with good results
Surgical techniques	
Gangliolysis	
Chemical	Alcohol previously used but could lead to cranial nerve damage. Phenol in glycerine or glycerine alone is less destructive. Glycerine may be useful for first division lesions, as results in less corneal anaesthesia
Radiofrequency	Large series show good long-term results. May be repeated
Balloon	May be as successful as other methods of gangliolysis. Extent of sensory loss not predictable

ATYPICAL FACIAL PAIN

DEFINITION

This is a vague term to describe a number of facial pain syndromes which do not fall into any other category. It was first coined to describe pains which did not respond to lesions of the trigeminal nerve, but it now represents a residual category for otherwise unclassifiable pains in the face. It probably includes a number of other related conditions, such as phantom tooth pain and atypical odontalgia. The clinical features are distinct from those of trigeminal neuralgia.

CLINICAL FEATURES

Patients have a mean age of 45, with a preponderance of females over males (82–100% in some series). Pain is characteristically burning or throbbing, continuous in nature, with no pain-free intervals. It is not usually related to any triggering stimulus. The pain usually starts in one quadrant of the mouth, but generally spreads and is often bilateral. It does not interfere with eating or sleeping. There is often a history of many previous dental extractions and procedures, nerve blocks and other attempts to relieve pain.

On examination there are few objective physical signs. Local tenderness is an inconsistent finding. Signs of autonomic dysfunction are notably absent.

AETIOLOGY

Almost by definition, no underlying pathophysiology can be determined. However, many of these patients present features of abnormal sensory processing which may be triggered by a previous minor injury or surgery. Patients with unilateral atypical facial pain (which is rarer than bilateral) may have an underlying organic pathology – possibly a migrainous type of condition. Relentlessly progressive symptoms should prompt exclusion of an underlying neoplasm. There are numerous anecdotal reports in the literature of cerebellopontine angle tumours presenting over a long period as atypical facial pain. Many authors consider atypical facial pain to be a 'psychiatric' condition, with depression being the most likely diagnosis.

MANAGEMENT

In general, surgical treatment and neuroablative procedures are contraindicated as they worsen symptoms.

Tricyclic antidepressants have a history of efficacy in this condition and have been demonstrated to be superior to placebo. The relief of pain seems to be independent of the antidepressant activity of the drug, and usual 'pain clinic' doses can be used. Atypical facial pain is one of the few conditions when the monoamine oxidase inhibitor class of antidepressants may be useful, often in conjunction with a small dose of phenothiazine.

Cognitive behavioural therapy is widely quoted as being successful.

CONCLUSION

Atypical facial pain is a rather meaningless diagnosis. Treatment is often unsatisfactory and patients will often continue to seek advice for alleviation of their pain.

TEMPOROMANDIBULAR JOINT PAIN

INTRODUCTION

The classification and nomenclature of disorders of the temporomandibular joint (TMJ) and masticatory muscles which present with pain have changed frequently in recent decades, largely with improvements in imaging techniques. Probably the most useful categorization divides TMJ disease into disorders of the masticatory muscles and problems arising from the TMJ (internal derangements and arthritis).

DISORDERS OF THE MASTICATORY MUSCLES

Conditions are variously described as TMJ myofascial pain dysfunction syndrome (TMP), facial arthromyalgia or TMJ dysfunction. Such disorders probably represent the majority of patients presenting to the pain relief clinic with TMJ pain.

INCIDENCE

Masticatory muscle dysfunction is common in the general population, with up to 50% of people experiencing problems at some time. Pain is a less common problem, occurring in around 10% of people. There are no differences in prevalence between the sexes or with increasing age. This contrasts with the statistics for those who seek treatment, where 80–90% of subjects present with pain, the majority are female (80%), and there is a tendency for symptoms to increase with age (except in the older elderly).

CLINICAL FEATURES

The pain is dull and aching in nature, arising in front of the ear and radiating to the temporal area and the angle of the mandible. There is occasional radiation to the neck. The pain may be bilateral. The temporal pattern of the pain varies but it is often worse on waking. Exacerbations may occur during eating.

On examination patients may have restricted mouth opening and tenderness to palpation of the masticatory muscles. Radiological investigation usually demonstrates no abnormality in the joint, although in the long term it may show some secondary changes.

AETIOLOGY

For many years occlusal disturbances were thought to be the cause of the pain, but it now appears that this is unlikely. Similarly, although bruxism may be associated with TMP the relationship is not thought to be causal. There seem to be considerable similarities between patients with fibromyalgia and those with TMP, which has led some authors to conclude that they are manifestations of the same condition. Present data suggest that derangement of the TMJ does not contribute significantly to the genesis of TMP, although interestingly there are a number of differences in the structure and function of the joint between males and females, which might suggest the apparent predisposition of females to TMP.

Conflicting data exist regarding the influence of psychological factors on TMP: in particular, sufferers do not differ from other pain patients or controls in premorbid personality type, response to illness or ability to cope with stress. The link between TMP and depression is also complex, and it is not clear whether any relationship observed suggests that depression is the cause or result of the pain. What is agreed is that the aetiology is generally multifactorial.

TREATMENT

Generally the management of TMP is conservative, with surgical options being reserved for those with disorders of the TMJ. Treatments are summarized in Table 20.2.

TABLE 20.2 Management of temporomandibular pain

Treatment	*Comments*
Reassurance and masticatory muscle exercise	Reduces subjective symptoms of dysfunction
Physical therapies (Trigger point injections, muscle stretch, heat and cold therapy)	Reduce muscle spasm
Occlusal splints	Good short-term response
Simple oral analgesics (NSAIDs, paracetamol)	Useful for acute exacerbations
Tricyclic antidepressants	Reported to produce significant pain relief
Behavioural management	Successful, with feedback and relaxation therapy particularly helpful
Acupuncture	More successful than placebo

INTERNAL DERANGEMENT OF THE TMJ AND TMJ ARTHRITIS

Internal derangement of the TMJ occurs when the relationship of the articular disc with the mandibular condyle is disturbed. It presents with pain, limited mouth opening and clicking or locking of the mandible. Previously diagnosed with arthrography, it is now more readily detected with MRI scanning. It is noteworthy that disc derangement is seen in normal (asymptomatic) subjects, and it is not clear whether surgery to reposition the disc is necessarily successful in reducing symptoms.

As with other synovial joints the TMJ is subject to degenerative arthritis, which presents as pain, stiffness on jaw movement and crepitus in the joint. Interestingly, such symptoms may resolve spontaneously, probably as a result of fibrocartilage degeneration. Management of these conditions is initially conservative, as for disorders of the masticatory muscles.

CHAPTER 21

CHRONIC PELVIC PAIN

INTRODUCTION

Persisting pelvic pain is common in women. Around half of gynaecological laparoscopies performed in the UK are for the investigation of pain. Attention is usually focused on the reproductive tract organs as the source, but it must be remembered that there are many urological, gastrointestinal and musculoskeletal conditions that present as pelvic pain. Patients who present to the pain clinic with chronic pelvic pain (CPP) will usually have had most of the common conditions excluded and will fall into the category of so-called chronic pelvic pain without obvious pathology. However, it is important to know the features of common causes of CPP.

GYNAECOLOGICAL CAUSES OF CPP

ENDOMETRIOSIS

Endometriosis (the presence of endometrium in sites other than the uterine cavity) can present in a variety of ways and may be an incidental finding at laparoscopy in asymptomatic individuals. The commonest presentation is that of pelvic pain, and it is found much more commonly at laparoscopy in those with pain than in those who are pain free.

Clinical symptoms correlate poorly with the extent of disease seen at laparoscopy. Treatment of the condition is both medical and surgical.

Medical treatments

These include:

- danazol – this has androgenic, antioestrogenic and antiprogestogenic activity. Generally, despite disease reduction, pain relief is disappointing. Androgenic side-effects are common
- gonadotrophin-releasing hormone analogues – these downregulate pituitary gonadotrophin secretion and can cause menopause-like side-effects.

Surgical treatment

In general there are few well conducted trials generating good outcome data. Surgical procedures include:

- laparoscopic excision/laser ablation of deposits
- total hysterectomy with bilateral salpingo-oophorectomy
- ablation of uterine nerves
- presacral neurectomy.

ADHESIONS

Peritoneal adhesions are found commonly at laparoscopy. They may arise as a result of endometriosis, infection (around 25% of women with pelvic inflammatory disease have pain) or previous surgery. It is not clear to what extent the findings at laparoscopy correlate with pain symptoms. Division of adhesions does not tend to produce long-lasting pain relief.

PELVIC CONGESTION

A large proportion of patients with CPP have evidence of dilated pelvic veins and congestion. This can be diagnosed at laparoscopy or, less invasively, with pelvic venography or ultrasound. It is postulated that venous stasis leads to local hypoxaemia and the release of pain-mediating chemicals.

Treatment with progestogens and gonadotrophin-releasing hormone analogues may be beneficial for pain resulting from pelvic congestion. Surgical management includes hysterectomy and salpingo-oophorectomy.

NON-GYNAECOLOGICAL CAUSES OF PELVIC PAIN

URINARY TRACT

Questions about urinary function should be part of the assessment of pelvic pain, i.e. ask about:

- urgency
- frequency
- hesitancy
- dysuria
- incomplete voiding.

In addition, cystourethroscopy should be considered in the investigation of CPP.

Common urinary tract causes of CPP and their management are summarized in Table 21.1.

GASTROINTESTINAL TRACT

A large proportion of CPP sufferers (7–60%), may have gastrointestinal disorders in particular irritable bowel syndrome (see p. 314). Diagnostic confusion arises because symptoms are exacerbated premenstrually, suggesting a gynaecological cause.

TABLE 21.1 Urinary causes of chronic pelvic pain and their management

Condition	*Management*
Acute/chronic infection	Antibiotics
Urethral syndrome (symptoms of irritation of the lower urinary tract – no cause found)	Modification of voiding habits Improvement of pelvic floor muscles Urethral dilatation Urethrotomy
Interstitial cystitis (chronic inflammation of the bladder)	Modification of voiding habits Bladder distension Tricyclic antidepressants

Features of irritable bowel syndrome

History
Colicky abdominal pain
Intermittent diarrhoea/constipation
Pain improves on bowel opening and worsens following food
Feeling of rectal fullness or incomplete evacuation
Symptoms of lower urinary tract irritation
Dyspareunia

Examination findings
Tenderness over sigmoid colon
Unusual discomfort on rectal examination
Pellet-like stools in rectum
NB: There tends to be coexisting psychopathology, e.g. somatization and anxiety disorders, depression and complaints about minor ailments.

Differential diagnosis
Inflammatory bowel disease
GI malignancy

Treatment
Medical treatment with anticholinergic drugs and bulk-forming agents.
Psychological support is important in this condition.

MUSCULOSKELETAL

Musculoskeletal problems may be the cause of CPP or may contribute to its symptomatology. Causes include lumbar spine disorders (see Chapter 16), muscle spasm of the pelvic floor (which may respond to physiotherapy, e.g. pelvic floor exercises) and abdominal wall pain. This latter category is quantitatively important in the pain clinic and can be divided into:

- scar pain (see Chapter 18)
- nerve entrapment
- muscular trigger points.

Nerve entrapment

There are two nerve entrapment syndromes which may present as CPP, ilioinguinal and abdominal.

Ilioinguinal nerve entrapment

The nerve arises from the L1 and L2 nerve roots, passes through the psoas and between quadratus lumborum and the parietal peritoneum and pierces the transversus abdominis medial to the iliac crest. It innervates the lower abdominal muscles, the skin of the groin and the base of the labia and inner thigh.

The nerve may be damaged at surgery (e.g. appendicectomy, Pfannenstiel incision, hernia repair), by direct trauma or by retraction of tissues. The pain tends to be stabbing in nature and exacerbated by exercise. Treatment is by single or repeated ilioinguinal nerve block using local anaesthetic and steroid. Some series report high success rates following surgical section of the nerve.

Abdominal cutaneous nerve entrapment

The nerves of the abdominal wall are the ventral rami of the lower six intercostal nerves and the first lumbar nerve. The lower five intercostal nerves pass between the transversus abdominis and internal oblique muscles and run into the rectus muscle. They supply and pierce the rectus and emerge through fascial tunnels at the lateral border of the rectus sheath to innervate the skin of the abdomen. They can become trapped or damaged following surgery, sudden movements or spontaneously.

The condition often presents as stabbing/pricking pain, worse on movement and on tensing the abdominal muscles, e.g. during coughing or sneezing. It may present as widespread right or left iliac fossa pain. On examination there is usually a marked trigger point at the lateral border of the rectus abdominis, exacerbated by lifting the head off the examination couch. Treatment is infiltration with local anaesthetic and steroid. More permanent pain relief may be achieved with cryotherapy or radiofrequency lesioning, or injection of phenol. It is important to identify the trigger point accurately before injection or lesioning.

Muscular trigger points

The abdominal wall is a common site for the development of muscle trigger points. A high proportion of patients with CPP have trigger points on the abdomen. These can be felt as nodules or bands within the muscle which are tender when compressed and may generate referred pain. Injection of local anaesthetic and steroid into accurately localized trigger points has a good success rate and injections may be repeated. If patients have a good but transient response, cryotherapy to the trigger point may provide lasting benefit. Other treatments, such as stretch and spray and TENS, have been described as successful.

PSYCHOLOGICAL FACTORS

Many patients with CPP have been seen by many specialists and been multiply investigated. Previously, absence of diagnosis led to the 'exclusion' diagnosis of 'psychogenic pain', but there is now a greater understanding of the role of psychological factors in a number of pain states. There have been many studies looking at the psychological characteristics of patients with CPP. Some series suggest that there is a higher incidence of depression in patients with CPP than in those without pelvic pain, but it is not clear whether psychological disturbance is a result of unremitting pain or precedes it. Figures are not available to compare features of depression between CPP and other chronic pain patients. Interestingly, the psychological profiles of women presenting with CPP are similar regardless of subsequent laparoscopic findings. It appears that CPP sufferers *may* show an increased incidence of somatization disorders, e.g. diarrhoea, constipation, dyspareunia, bloating and nausea. The relationship with irritable bowel syndrome has been discussed.

Data from the USA suggest that there seems to be an increased incidence of physical and/or sexual abuse in sufferers of CPP, and patients with such a history may be refractory to treatment.

As with other chronic pain states, an integrated medical (including surgical) and psychological approach to management is likely to be successful. It is important to take serious note of the patient's complaint, explain fully any underlying pathology and that complete cure may be an unrealistic goal. Relaxation training and the teaching of strategies to avoid or reduce pain are likely to be helpful. Of most benefit are multidisciplinary pain management programmes.

CONCLUSION

Pelvic pain is common and has a disruptive effect on patients' relationships and sexual function. Although it is important to understand the many conditions that may present with pelvic pain, the aetiology is often multifactorial and assessment and management by a multidisciplinary team is likely to produce the most satisfactory outcome.

SECTION 5

PSYCHOLOGY AND PAIN

CHAPTER 22

PSYCHOLOGY AND PAIN

PSYCHOLOGY

Psychology is the academic study of mind and behaviour in a social context. Research and practice in pain is informed largely by experimental, clinical and health branches of psychology. Experimental psychology explores the basic cognitive, behavioural, physiological and pharmacological mechanisms that underpin a pain experience. Clinical and health psychology are concerned with understanding why pain and suffering are exacerbated or maintained, and with ameliorating the suffering associated with pain.

PSYCHOLOGICAL FACTORS IN PAIN PERCEPTION AND COMPLAINT

The definition of pain has at its centre the importance of psychological factors. It is clear that the pain experience has sensory, affective and evaluative components. Undue focus upon any one of these areas increases the margin of error in both diagnosis and treatment. The affective and evaluative components can be understood as psychological. All will be implicated in presentation and treatment.

Anxiety

Pain is closely related to fear, both being processed in older (subcortical) brain systems. Anger and fear are a common corollary of any pain experience. Fear processes are biologically useful and adaptive, serving as a protective warning system. However, we learn to control fear in situations where aggression or flight would be inappropriate, but many people develop specific fears known as 'phobias', and others develop more generalized anxieties. Both acute and chronic pain are often exacerbated by anxiety.

Phobias

Phobias of wasps, spiders and heights are common complaints in the general population. However rational one can be about a feared object, the **experience** is one of intense fear and an overwhelming desire for escape. Other common phobias are of needles, hospitals and blood. Reactions to these can be strong, such as fainting and sudden intense muscle tension. Specific phobias are easily treatable and one should refer to a clinical psychologist.

Generalized anxiety disorder (GAD)

Some people develop a disorder of general attention which is best characterized by a heightened awareness and judgement of personal threat. Such people are in a state of readiness, are highly distractible, and have concentration and memory difficulties. In such a state information loss is highly likely. GAD is very common and can be treated. Most of us will meet the criteria for this at some time, especially during stressful events such as examinations. Chronic GAD requires a referral to a clinical psychologist.

Acute pain and anxiety

Anxiety functions to protect us by priming our senses to recognize any threat so that we can respond more quickly. Just as a wasp phobic will hear the buzzing of a wasp before a non-phobic, so a person fearing pain will feel pain more quickly and in many cases more intensely than a person not fearing pain. This effect is robust across pain conditions. The more anxious the patient about an impending painful procedure the greater the pain reported and the longer the recovery time.

Chronic pain and anxiety

Those with chronic pain typically have some degree of allodynia and hyperalgesia. Part of this increased likelihood to report increased pain can be understood as a perceptual habit which has its origins in fear processes. Increased anxiety increases pain, and more pain is anxiety provoking. In chronic pain this often forms a vicious circle, dependent upon the meaning of the pain. If the pain is unpredictable and provokes fears of life-threatening disease patients often become clinically anxious (as in the case of fibromyalgia). Where the fear is one of damage to a specific area, the patient often avoids stressing that area (as in back pain). This typically leads to a disuse syndrome.

Depression

Depression is a common complaint in the general population. Although we all report periods of depressed mood, clinical depression is best represented by an overwhelming nihilism and intense apathy. There is an association between pain and depression. Those who are depressed often report muscle pain and fatigue. Head pain is also a common complaint of depression. Where depression is associated with acute pain it will normally be unrelated but will worsen the pain and slow recovery. Those who are extremely depressed often report a perceptual numbness and an absence of pain complaint to injury or to procedural pain.

Depression and chronic pain

Chronic pain was for some time thought to be a variant of depressive illness; however, no evidence for this causal association has been found. Similarly, there is no evidence that a tendency to depression is a risk factor for acute pains becoming chronic. Depression is now understood to be a reaction to the extensively disabling effects of chronic pain. This can affect not only the patient but the family, friends, carers and physicians. It fuels a helplessness and a hopelessness, a loss of self-esteem and a loss of confidence.

Anger and hostility

This is common in chronic pain and is characterized by impatience, a focus on singular goals and a quickness to argument. Anger is very distressing for patients, is associated with lack of control over the pain and treatment, fuels depression and often ends in hostile communication. Such hostility functions to isolate the patient further, thereby increasing depression and pain.

Pain behaviour

Behaviour is a form of communication. We learn how to behave and the parameters of appropriate and inappropriate behaviour from social interaction. The focus on behaviour in pain research and treatment arose from a concern with the social factors that exacerbate and maintain chronic pain. A pain behaviour such as a grimace communicates distress and is likely to produce sympathetic behaviours from others. This is perfectly normal. It is argued that dangers arise when sympathetic or helpful behaviours become reinforcing of complaint and serve to exacerbate pain.

In trying to make sense of seemingly strange pain behaviour it is important to remember that:

- there is no objective measure of the normality of pain behaviour because there is no objective test for pain
- there is also no simple relationship between damage and pain. Minor damage can cause intense pain and major damage can cause mild pain
- given central mechanisms and descending inhibition, pain amplification is common in clinical settings
- there is no evidence for the existence of a pain personality
- we are generally unaware of what our behaviour communicates to others.

The normality of pain behaviour is defined by the situation in which the pain is observed and the responses of observers to the behaviour. Where pain is seen to be *inappropriate* this is normally *inappropriate* to the physician's understanding of what should occur. Chronic pain patients will demonstrate extreme chronic pain behaviour where the following reinforcements are present:

- where pain is central to communication (e.g. to receive a diagnosis or treatment)
- where the person is fearful of increased pain (e.g. in straight leg raising)
- where the meaning of pain is fear inducing
- where there is an absence of reinforcement for non-pain communications.

With chronic pain this last aspect is possibly the most important. The focus on the pain behaviour construct has rightly taught that excessive sympathy and solicitousness can exacerbate suffering, disability and dependency. Just as important is the lack of reward patients receive for other aspects of daily life that non-pain sufferers take for granted. It is in this way that patients can become pain focused. Other aspects of life receive scant attention, and where this is forthcoming it is rarely positive.

Cognitive style

Cognition is a general term for 'thought'. The focus on the thoughts associated with pain is of central importance to understanding why pain experiences vary so much. Certain styles of cognition have been studied in situations of acute and chronic pain.

Self-efficacy

This refers to the beliefs we all have about our ability to change our lives. Those in chronic pain often develop a low self-efficacy. This is due to the experience of treatments over which control is taken by powerful others, and is also a factor of depression and fear. It has been shown to account for the failure of certain physical treatments and is critically important in the maintenance of any change brought about in hospital settings. However useful a physical treatment may be, if a person has no belief in their own ability to effect it, it will ultimately fail.

Attribution of causality

We need to make sense of experience. This is of crucial importance in pain settings. Because pain is most often understood as a symptom of something it is often highly anxiety provoking, and patients will ruminate and fantasize as to the cause of the pain. This is perfectly normal. We need to make sense of pain. Although many pains can be made sense of, dangers arise in the pain clinic, where many chronic pains are senseless and pointless. Chronic pain patients often desire meaning for their pain and are not easily reassured (see below): most attribute the cause of their pain to a physical disorder. Although pain patients often score highly on measures of hypochondriacal thinking, primary hypochondriasis is extremely rare in chronic pain populations.

Attribution of blame

Apart from the the need to make sense of pain and its cause, many patients often demonstrate a need to attribute blame or responsibility for the pain. Although this is a fairly under-researched area, in chronic pain such cognitions are clinically important. Many chronic pain patients show high levels of immiserating guilt and shame as they blame themselves for the changes in their lives and those around them. Other chronic pain patients demonstrate anger and anxiety at those believed to have caused the pain, those who may have treated and/or those who may have refused to treat. Again, these patterns of thinking often exacerbate suffering and hamper change.

Catastrophizing

This particular pattern of thinking or cognitive style has been identified as a risk factor for chronic pain. It also explains the largest amount of variance in the outcome of treatments in chronic pain: those who are high catastrophizers fare worse in physical and behavioural rehabilitation. A catastrophizing cognitive style is one in which the consequences of events are quickly and anxiously blown out of proportion. A typical example would be the patient who says: 'This is not going to get better, it can only get worse – and then what's going to happen? It's bound to spread, I'm never going to get better, I'll lose my job, my wife will leave me – I can't see any end to this. You've got to help me doctor.'

THE PSYCHOLOGY OF THE PAIN CONSULTATION

The tools of psychology are words and interpretation. How we come to understand health and illness is through what is said, shown and demonstrated. Equally important is what is not said, what is omitted, what is thought and feared but never asked. This section addresses underlying ideas and issues in the pain consultation and some of the guiding principles for interaction in the consultation process.

Pain does not always mean damage

Where we interact with patients it is normally in the context of an extreme stress, such as intense pain, the threat of intense pain, or disability. In this interaction much is assumed and unspoken. Most importantly, it is commonly assumed that the pain must mean damage. We are trained to understand pain as a 'symptom' of disorder. It demands that we investigate, diagnose and treat. Patients will understand this. It is important to remember that the patient who is thought to be responsible in this setting is the one who reports (as objectively as possible) upon somatic events in order to aid diagnosis or treatment. As the patient role is a passive one, this leads to much information loss, a lack of clarity about details, unspoken questions and a poor learning environment for the doctor.

When the pain is not useful diagnostically (as in the case of chronic benign pains) this can often lead to a confusion and a breakdown in trust in the doctor–patient relationship. Patients may continue to offer information for investigation, often to the frustration of the physician. The absence of a diagnosis may be understood by the patient to mean incompetence by the hospital or doctor. Equally the failure of the pain to be related to any identifiable physical or pharmacological process often leaves the physician with no other solution but to 'leap to the head' for an explanation, as one becomes suspicious that perhaps the patient is mentally unstable. When pain does not make sense, the patient can quickly be seen as 'mad' and the doctor 'bad'.

The only solution is to remember that there is ample evidence for the lack of association between pain and injury. The patient needs an understanding of their pain that does not implicate them in its production. One must take time to explain why pain without identifiable damage can occur.

Pain and suffering are always underestimated

We consistently underestimate the intensity of pain compared to the judgement of the patient. This is a common and robust finding. There are two areas where this is particularly extensive:

- *Pain in children.* It was once thought that neonates and infants did not feel pain to the same extent as adults. Recent evidence shows this to be false: children do suffer pain. Despite this, children are routinely under-medicated and are often not offered any form of analgesia. This may be due to exaggerated and unsubstantiated fears of addiction on the part of the prescribing physician. One should remember that addiction is a contextual affect: addiction to medication given in acute settings is a rare occurrence. More often children are under-medicated because of communication problems. Where a child cannot communicate pain, parents and carers also underestimate the amount of pain suffered (see Measures, below).
- *Myth of acceptable pain.* There is a prevalent idea that some pain is expected and therefore not a priority for analgesia. Common examples are postoperative pain, procedural pain (e.g. heel lancing, injection pain) and cancer pain. In fact, much of this pain can be effectively ameliorated if it is seen as a problem. This myth is common to both patients and practitioners. Patients will often not communicate distress directly, as they expect pain and discomfort. Under-medicated, this leads to protracted recovery periods.

Measuring pain and its effects

Measurement is everything in pain and pain relief. There is an academic and a clinical industry dedicated to the production of questionnaires and scales. As pain is fundamentally subjective and not open to objective validation it is ethically difficult to question the report of a patient's experience. However, pain is a complex event and most patients find it difficult to communicate effectively the extent of their perception.

Common measures

The most commonly employed measures are unidimensional analogue scaling techniques. The ubiquitous visual analogue scale (VAS) is merely a 10 cm line anchored by the words 'worst imaginable pain' and 'no pain'. Patients are required to mark a cross over the line between the two anchor points to express the intensity of the pain. Other VASs of mood and disability are also commonly used. The benefit of these measures is that they are quick and easy to administer and have some validity. They are less useful in research settings, where precision is required and more information needed. Other common measures are the McGill Pain Questionnaire (Chapter 9), which attempts to capture the multidimensional aspects of the pain. It is well validated and reliable. There is also a short form of this scale.

Non-pain measures

In most cases the measurement of pain is not sufficient. Pain, even very short-lived pain, affects mood, cognition, function and beliefs about illness and recovery. In chronic pain conditions it is often only one of many important treatment objects. In chronic pain efforts should be made to assess function, anxiety, depressive status, beliefs about treatment and expectations of the treatment process. Well validated and reliable measures exist for these dimensions of pain, but visual analogue scales can easily be made if others cannot be found. Often a treatment may not affect pain, but rather decrease suffering via changes in mood or function. This can often be missed in clinical settings.

Children's pain measures

For children under the age of 4 one needs to observe behavioural changes. These include withdrawal, avoidance, 'pain face', crying, holding, irritability, food refusal, not playing and poor attention. These do not always signify pain but are often present with pain. For 4–5-year-olds the 'pieces of hurt' method is recommended. Give the child five poker chips, play bricks or stones and tell them that each chip is a piece of hurt, where one piece means a little hurt and two pieces mean more hurt. Then ask the child how many 'pieces of hurt' he or she feels. Children over 5 also respond well to visual scales, such as face scales. These are available from the literature. Children over 10 can often use VAS measures, or can be asked how bad their pain is on a scale of 0–10, where 0 is no pain and 10 is the worst pain possible.

Analgesia and suffering can be improved with instruction

Where effective forms of analgesia are available they can be strengthened by a number of techniques of psychological delivery. Where pharmacological therapies are not indicated, psychological techniques should be used.

Information about pain

Information about the impending pain of a procedure can crucially affect the experience. Information about the time course of a pain is effective in reducing suffering and complaint. As a general rule, people can cope with many sensory aversive events if they know how long they are going to last. Information about the sensations of the pain (e.g. pricking, burning, thumping) is less useful but can also help the patient gain a sense of control over the experience. Equally important with the chronic pain patient is honesty about the cause of the pain. Telling someone in the pain clinic that pain is very unlikely ever to go away is a crucial first step to rehabilitation.

Information about illness

Problems of miscommunication surround the issue of diagnosis and treatment plans. Common phrases can set the catastrophizing (see above) patient into a persistent worry. For example, as a physician one may wish to explain fully to a patient the X-ray of the spine. Pointing to the 'degenerative disc disease', for example, as something 'not to worry about' often reappears 6 months later in the pain clinic as 'the doctor told me I had a crumbling spine'. As a further example, many chronic pain patients are confused by the idea of a 'flare' in pain, as this word seems to communicate a disease process that may not be warranted.

Cognitive coping techniques

Many of us routinely use thinking techniques to reduce pain. One should remember that a preferred technique is normally better than a taught one. With procedural pain, for example, some people prefer to distract themselves for the entire procedure, whereas others benefit from being informed about each detail. Distraction techniques can be useful and are most effective when the patient uses something personally meaningful for them, something that is complex and detailed but has structure. The best form of distraction is probably storytelling or daydreaming. Children are often able to use these techniques more effectively than adults.

Relaxation

This refers to an enforced state of deep relaxation rather than everyday time out. People can be taught to relax prior to stressful medical events or procedures. The common example of this is the widespread success of Lamaze training for parturition pain. Relaxation can be taught in a number of ways. All involve deep and slow breathing. The popular method is deep muscle relaxation, which involves the systematic tensing and untensing of muscles to learn the feeling of becoming physically relaxed. Other methods include the use of imagery and mild hypnotic suggestion. All are affective in increasing analgesia and positively affect recovery time. It is, however, time-consuming to train patients in their use. Not all health professionals are skilled in training. Be aware that sudden deep relaxation can be frightening for some people.

Guidelines for treating those in pain

- Find a quiet place that will aid communication and reduce anxiety. Avoid interruption from other staff, as this will break any trust in communication.
- Give a clear time-frame for the course of the pain and the course of the analgesia. If there is a large range then give the approximate figures and the range.

- Explain clearly what the patient may reliably expect to feel (e.g. sleepy and dry mouthed). Where side-effects are indicated, explain that one has to give such information (as a pilot would talk about 'in the event of an emergency').
- Always take a measure of pain and distress.
- Assess normal coping techniques, e.g. What do you do when you go to the dentist or have an injection? Suggest some mental techniques in line with these.
- If there is time (e.g. prior to a painful procedure such as debridement) then refer the patient to the hospital pain team or, in their absence, a psychologist for preparation (including relaxation training).
- Remember that there will be a small proportion of people who have psychological issues more encompassing than the pain (such as clinical fear or depression) for whom the opinion of a clinical psychologist should be sought.

THE PSYCHOLOGIST IN THE PAIN CLINIC

Where pain response teams exist they typically involve a pain psychologist or have had input from one in their development. However, most pain psychologists will be based in the pain clinic. How a psychologist works in the pain clinic is entirely dependent upon the team. Psychologists can work directly with patients, with groups of patients, or as a part of the team, working through other health professionals. The three most common ways that a psychologist works are:

- joint consultation/assessment of complex chronic pain problems
- with individuals or with a family
- directing and delivering cognitive behavioural therapy for pain management.

Joint consultation/assessment of complex pain problems

By far the majority of the work of the psychologist in the pain clinic will be with the complex adult chronic pain patient. However, it is increasingly common for a psychologist to work as part of the pain team, or as a specialist in oncology, paediatrics or other specialties. Where possible the psychologist should assess the patient with the consultant physician. The psychologist would normally be concerned to assess the extent of disability due to pain, and to minimally intervene with an explanation of the process of becoming disabled by the pain. Working in partnership with the physician adds credibility and trust to the consultation and offers a means to address miscommunications. It also provides a rich ground for cross-professional education. Although there will be issues particular to individual patients, the psychological assessment of the pain patient will typically include:

- the patient's understanding of the causes of the pain
- the language used in describing the sensation, location and duration of pain
- the extent of pain behaviour
- the patient's understanding of current or suggested treatment plans
- the effect of pain on everyday life
- the effect of pain on sleeping patterns
- the effect of pain on family relations
- the effect of pain on isolation and social responsiveness
- current and recent depression
- current and recent risk of suicide
- the extent of anxiety processes in the exacerbation of suffering
- problem-solving skills and the effects of failed attempts at coping
- the ability to think of the future and change
- the treatment wishes of the patient and others involved in care.

A treatment plan will then be jointly agreed with the patient, the physician and the psychologist, that would include the results of the above. Common issues in chronic pain that may be addressed at this stage by the psychologist are:

- confusion about conflicting advice and the meaning of medical terminology
- confusion about medication use (e.g. the use of amytriptiline as an analgesic)
- fear of addiction and fear of increased pain on medication withdrawal
- difficulty in believing that no curative treatment is available
- unrealistic expectations of treatments and possible change
- fear of approaching change and rehabilitation
- lack of trust in health professionals
- anger and depression at lack of control over pain
- fear of blame and dismissal as being 'mad'
- readiness to approach rehabilitation
- adjustment to loss of identity as healthy.

Working individually or with a family

There are a number of reasons for working individually with a patient, with couples or with a family group. Working with children with pain, for example, nearly always means also working with care givers or family members. Although many children are seen by psychologists in child and family therapy centres, there is a growing recognition for the need of specialist pain psychology for children.

Common interventions are for dealing with painful procedures, such as venipuncture, plaster removal etc. Often this is where fear is paramount and other pain relief measures cannot be used. Similar techniques of pain relief and anxiety reduction are also commonly used for postoperative pain and distress. Other members of the ward team can be trained in these. Children also suffer from chronic pain problems. A child pain psychologist may expect to see children who are having difficulty coping with the pain of juvenile rheumatoid arthritis, or juvenile fibromyalgia, or other musculoskeletal pains. A common reason for referral to a child psychologist is for abdominal pain, which often presents as a result of other problems, such as children refusing to go to school. A common chronic pain problem seen is in those with migraine, where again the psychologist would work to help the child predict the triggers for attacks and provide non-pharmacological methods of relief.

Many of the issues that are pertinent to adult pain are also relevant to children's pain. In particular there is often a problem with children not feeling believed about their pain. This can often be exacerbated by school refusal and the absence of objective physical markers (e.g. in recurrent abdominal pain). Special consideration is given in the assessment of children in pain to:

- effects of their pain upon siblings, parents and care givers
- effects on their schooling and learning
- effects on their mental health of persistent doubt and blame
- family functioning and the place of pain in the family's communication
- parent helplessness and parental control
- children's beliefs about pain (in particular the effects of fantastical thinking).

Child clinical psychologists need always to be called earlier rather than later. Often their intervention is most clearly understood when a child is markedly distressed. However, there is excellent evidence for the effectiveness of psychological strategies in the prevention of pain and distress. Similarly, effective psychological therapies for children are often best delivered in a partnership with other paediatric health workers.

Some adults with chronic pain may also have more complex psychological mediators of their disability, in addition to persistent pain. A psychologist in the pain clinic will, upon occasion, decide that the patient is best treated with a partner, as a family or alone, depending upon the presentation. It is not uncommon for brief individual psychotherapeutic interventions to be used within a wider pain-related treatment plan. Where long-term psychotherapy is indicated this should ideally be addressed outside the pain clinic.

Where patients are suitable for cognitive behavioural intervention (see below) but are not willing or able to cope with a group environment, this can also be delivered on an individual basis. The benefits of this are that the therapy can be tailored more directly to the individual and their pace of change. Not available to use are the powerful modelling effects of other people with pain changing their ideas and behaviours during the therapy.

Directing and delivering cognitive behavioural therapy for pain management

Cognitive behavioural therapy is an approach to rehabilitation that takes full account of the patterns of thinking that exacerbate and maintain pain and disability. Also used is the understanding of the patterns and habits that people fall into where others respond to support illness or ignore non-pain activities. At time of writing there are 34 randomized controlled trials showing that cognitive behavioural therapy is effective in its main goals of:

- decreasing disability
- increasing function
- reducing medication
- reducing the need for hospital medicine
- reducing anxiety
- reducing depression
- increasing independence
- increasing problem-solving skills.

This therapy should be delivered by a multidisciplinary team of health professionals as a cohesive programme. Ideally teams should have the input of the psychologist, the physician, the physiotherapist, an occupational therapist and a nurse. All team members must have been trained in pain management skills. The therapy is delivered in both outpatient and in-patient settings.

Outpatient programmes

These are more educational in nature and focus on training individuals in the skills needed for coping with pain, including:

- relaxation training
- thought stopping or challenging
- discussion of pain behaviours with families
- pain education
- pacing activities and setting achievable goals
- dealing with setbacks when they occur
- sleep management.

These are often delivered for two afternoons a week (or less) over a 6–8-week period. Not all outpatient programmes are alike. Most include elements of education and relaxation, but many differ to the extent to which they deliver cognitive therapies or focus on behavioural change. The role of the psychologist here would be in jointly assessing patients for their suitability for such interventions. They would also be responsible for the delivery and coherence of such a therapy.

Inpatient programmes

Where patients are admitted for cognitive behavioural pain management this is usually to a non-clinical, hotel-like environment. Efforts are made to provide as non-medical or illness-free an environment as possible. Many patients entering in-patient cognitive behavioural pain management are too disabled for outpatient services, or are in need of a more thorough approach than the skills-based model can provide. The UK in-patient programmes are of either 3 or 4 weeks in duration. In-patient settings offer more opportunity for addressing the behavioural factors that are implicated in maintained disability. More emphasis is placed on a structured cognitive therapeutic intervention and greater opportunities are available to coordinate aspects of the therapy into a coherent whole. More emphasis is normally placed on including significant other people in the therapy, and on how to continue the rehabilitation once the patient is returned to the home setting.

As polymedication is a significant problem in chronic pain, inpatient programmes would also include detoxification programmes. There are also more opportunities to work with setbacks in the rehabilitation.

As there is a growing recognition of the importance of psychological factors in the development of chronic pain, more psychologists are working with primary care physicians to provide secondary preventative methods to stop acute pain from becoming chronic.

CONCLUSION

Psychology is an everyday reality in the treatment of pain. It is possible to increase or ameliorate the pain and the suffering associated with it by the way in which treatments are delivered. There are also specific therapies that can be offered by trained psychologists. Psychologists are trained as consultants who are able to offer expertise in assessment and therapy. They can also increase the effectiveness of other therapies, working as core members of a pain treatment facility or team within a larger centre.

INDEX